BIG
&
BOLD:

Yoga for the Plus-Size Woman

■ ■ ■

Laura Burns

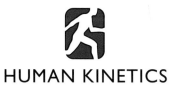

HUMAN KINETICS

Library of Congress Cataloging-in-Publication Data

Names: Burns, Laura, 1982- author.
Title: Big & bold : yoga for the plus-size woman / Laura Burns.
Other titles: Big and bold
Description: Champaign, IL : Human Kinetics, [2022]
Identifiers: LCCN 2021010201 (print) | LCCN 2021010202 (ebook) | ISBN
  9781718200098 (paperback) | ISBN 9781718200104 (epub) | ISBN
  9781718200111 (pdf)
Subjects: LCSH: Hatha yoga--Popular works. | Women--Health and hygiene.
Classification: LCC RA781.7 .B867 2022 (print) | LCC RA781.7 (ebook) |
  DDC 613.7/046--dc23
LC record available at https://lccn.loc.gov/2021010201
LC ebook record available at https://lccn.loc.gov/2021010202

ISBN: 978-1-7182-0009-8 (print)

Senior Acquisitions Editor: Michelle Maloney; **Senior Developmental Editor:** Cynthia McEntire; **Managing Editor:** Hannah Werner; **Copyeditor:** Amy Pavelich; **Permissions Manager:** Martha Gullo; **Senior Graphic Designer:** Joe Buck; **Cover Designer:** Keri Evans; **Cover Design Specialist:** Susan Rothermel Allen; **Photograph (cover):** Shannon Cottrell / Human Kinetics, Inc.; **Photographs (interior):** Shannon Cottrell; **Photo Production Specialist:** Amy M. Rose; **Photo Production Manager:** Jason Allen; **Printer:** Versa Press

We thank Still Yoga in Silverlake, California, for assistance in providing the location for the photo shoot for this book. We also thank Natalie Dunbar for modeling at the photo shoot.

Human Kinetics books are available at special discounts for bulk purchase. Special editions or book excerpts can also be created to specification. For details, contact the Special Sales Manager at Human Kinetics.

Printed in the United States of America   10 9 8 7 6 5 4 3 2 1

The paper in this book is certified under a sustainable forestry program.

Human Kinetics
1607 N. Market Street
Champaign, IL 61820
USA

United States and International
Website: **US.HumanKinetics.com**
Email: info@hkusa.com
Phone: 1-800-747-4457

Canada
Website: **Canada.HumanKinetics.com**
Email: info@hkcanada.com

E8151

Tell us what you think!
Human Kinetics would love to hear what we
can do to improve the customer experience.
Use this QR code to take our brief survey.

With gratitude for all the beautiful souls who've trusted me as their teacher and taught me so much. In solidarity with anyone who has ever felt disconnected from their body. May we all experience the freedom and autonomy that come from embodiment and body liberation.

CONTENTS

Part I   Set for Success

Chapter 1   Start With Confidence! 3

It can be intimidating for folks in larger bodies to think about trying yoga, because often it seems like the world of yoga isn't made for them. This chapter will help you choose the right style of yoga for your needs, get you ready to try out classes or create your own home practice, and offer plus-size-specific insights to help you feel empowered and confident.

Chapter 2   Get Your Gear 19

Let's talk yoga props and activewear! What do you actually need for a strong and supported practice? Where can you find the best gear? How do you decide from among the many options? As a beginner, you may feel like you need to gather every potentially useful prop. Skip being overwhelmed—streamline your practice with only the tools you actually need.

Part II   Get Moving

Chapter 3   Warming Up and Breathing Exercises 37

Gentle warm-up exercises and basic breathing techniques form the foundation of your yoga practice. Learn various ways to sit comfortably on the floor, move safely from standing to seated, prepare the body for practice, and use breath to cultivate the mood or energy you need in your day.

Chapter 4   Seated and Kneeling Poses 61

Embrace the freedom and accessibility that seated and kneeling poses bring to your practice. You can stretch and strengthen your body from a seated or kneeling position and create both relaxing and challenging practices to fit your needs.

Chapter 5   Standing Poses 89

Explore the world of standing postures and find balance, strength, flexibility, and mind–body connection. You can find stability and support with props, and the many options for body alignment will allow you to experience standing poses in ways that work for your body.

POSE FINDER

RECLINED POSES

RESTORATIVE POSES

ENERGIZING PRACTICES

RELAXING PRACTICES

SERIES PREFACE

I'm going to say it: *Fitness* is a loaded word.

My Amazonian body won me gold ribbons, crossed the finish line first in races, was awarded a coveted athletic scholarship to Syracuse, and led what began as a personal passion into a global movement for inclusive beauty decades ago.

For me, being fit is a source of joy and accomplishment. It's in my blood. I get out a few times each week and every weekend to smell the air and put miles under my feet. The more time I'm in nature during every season, the happier I am.

My commitment to living a fit lifestyle is nonnegotiable, even if I don't fit the cultural ideal of what healthy or fit looks like. But millions of women face judgment, a disparaging word, or a disapproving glance, especially when a gleeful, confident, and curvy bod announces her triathlon goals or athletic accomplishment on an IG feed or—God forbid—skips by in real time.

It seriously makes me wonder: Why do happy, fit, and curvy people piss so many off, and why is *fit* a term for a select few?

No, my sweaty, joyous souls; fitness includes all body shapes, ages, and sizes! The Cooper Institute in Dallas tapped into this years ago when their data and research reflected an array of body types, not just the very thin, that could (and do) achieve fitness. Being fit is something all of us can set as a goal and attain, regardless of size.

Why on earth should only a few folks be able to claim a fit and healthy life? We all come in various shapes and sizes—be it tall and angular, naturally muscular, or naturally curvier. When we add our skeletal structures for each body type (i.e., XS, S, M, L, XL, XXL, XXXL), there's a bouquet of human expression going on that includes those embracing a fit lifestyle. When I break down who we are in this way, it makes sense to me and allows me to be who I am and not try to be what I'm not. Fitness is a journey open and available to all shapes and sizes (and ages)!

But how do we hold on to this inclusive mindset?

First, your purse is your power tool. Ignore marketing designed to motivate a purchase and make companies a lot of money. Second, don't buy into false beliefs that fitness, beauty, and success are an exclusive membership for the select few. It's time to get off the never-ending hamster wheel fueled by self-defeating diets and the mindset of "fitting in" and ask yourself, "For what?"

We're all in this together for goodness' sake, and I've got a news flash—this is *so* not a size thing; it's a women's rights issue. I beg you: Get off that train to nowhere *now* and allow yourself to be totally absorbed in the magic within the pages of this book. They will set you free from body bashing, comparisons, and put-downs and set you in a new direction of self-discovery that you never thought possible. All it takes is one step, then another, then another, and you're off enjoying *your* fitness journey.

Start by creating your own story. Be your own sweaty badass babe rocking life, no matter what. Own it and claim *you*! Once you drop the mic on limiting beliefs, others will wonder where all your fabulousness is coming from and become curious about the miracles being performed in your life. Start; you'll see. Dance, swim, glide, ride, walk, run, and sway; allow various forms of movement to flow through you as your new self-expression.

Above all, by engaging in our own fitness routines for the sheer joy of play as if our lives depend on it, we unleash our very own superpower to be fit under our terms, regardless of our size. Our glorious, magnificent, and powerful body pumps blood every day without being told to do so and allows us to live this incredible life. Honor it by slowing down to listen to it. Once we become our own body's bodyguard, the stars align and a path is cleared to a life *we* get to choose.

Fitness is by no means a race to the fittest; it's a lifestyle. With intention. A life committed to joy, wellness, and getting a kick out of being fit. I'm excited for you. An empowering new frame of mind around fitness is awaiting you here.

In joy,
xo
Emme
#playsweatwin

PREFACE

Those who know me now would be surprised to learn that I spent a large portion of my life as a yoga hater. Really! Not only was I not a fan of yoga, but I went out of my way to make sure everyone knew it. Friends knew my arguments almost by heart. I made fun of yoga postures and rued the day I'd ever stepped foot on a yoga mat. I was convinced that yoga was for a type of person that I'd never be, and I felt compelled to tell everyone how much I disliked everything about the practice.

But let's back up and give you some context about this negative mindset I had about yoga. Growing up as the fat* kid in every class, I learned from an early age how to defend my heart and mind from bullies and well-meaning, but offensive, strangers. This defense mechanism really came into play when teenage Laura Burns attempted to try this yoga thing that so many of her friends loved. On the advice from *so many friends*, I signed up for a Bikram yoga class. Are you laughing yet? If you're not familiar with the name Bikram yoga, perhaps you've heard of hot yoga? Yes, they mean *hot*—really, really hot! If the one piece of advice you take away from this book is this, I consider my job done: Don't take a hot yoga class as your first introduction to yoga! Learn from my mistake and spare yourself the agony of a combination of not knowing what to do with your body, having an instructor obviously not know what to do with your body, and being the sweatiest you've ever been in your life in a steamy room full of other hot and *fragrant* people.

So, is it any wonder I hated yoga? I tried class after class of different styles of yoga, but each time was the same experience: I would come to class optimistic and anxious, find that my teacher didn't know how to teach my larger body, be ignored or overly highlighted by the instructor, and leave feeling like a failure and sure that yoga just wasn't meant for a body like mine. After a handful of experiences like this, I became a yoga hater and vowed never to step on a mat again! I stuck to that and stayed away from anything yoga related for a decade. I rebuffed my friends' attempts to get me to join their studio or even to practice in their home with a video.

Unfortunately, I had a negative introduction to the world of yoga and let it color my perception for a long time. I was shown and truly believed that yoga was not for folks in larger bodies, and I am so grateful to now realize that's wrong. The silver lining to my story is that I did finally find the resources and tools I needed to make yoga work for me and the body I have today, and, from there, my life completely changed. I'm so excited to bring these resources and tools to you in the hopes that your life can change as well!

*You will notice that I refer to myself as a *fat* person, rather than using a euphemism such as *curvy, plus-sized,* or *fluffy.* This is how I feel comfortable referring to myself, but I will use *plus-sized* throughout the book to refer to other bodies.

"WAIT—WHO ARE YOU?"

You might be wondering, *Who the heck is this former yoga hater?* I am a fat woman, perpetual student of yoga, and believer in the power and wonder of joyful movement in all forms, and I am firmly in favor of larger-bodied folks making yoga a part of their daily lives. I studied hatha yoga (more on this later) with an emphasis on creating gentle postures with varying levels of support and accessible challenges. I teach classes, workshops, and continuing education training around the United States for students and teachers looking to find ways to incorporate body liberation and empowerment into their practices.

I've always been very active, participating in dance, swimming, running, and hiking. I love these forms of movement and have always practiced them as a fat person. I never thought of my size as limiting my ability to participate in anything I wanted to try. Unfortunately, other people often saw me differently than I saw myself. This kind of weight stigma sometimes made being part of a team or group unpleasant, which caused me to push myself harder than I should have as a means of proving myself to those who doubted my capability. Finally finding the benefits of yoga was a revelation that truly changed the way I engage with my body and with movement in general! My yoga practice meets me where I am at that moment and provides both mental and physical benefits that help me to stay grounded, centered, and embodied. Unlike other movement forms, yoga encourages me to release my tendency to push and potentially injure myself in an attempt to prove that I am as good and worthy as the thin people around me. My practice is a conversation with myself and is not affected by the strength or skill of anyone else. I no longer feel the need to be validated by others! This internal focus fits so beautifully with the body-positive work I've done to combat the body shame and oppression I've lived with all my life.

If you're reading this book, you're likely also a larger-bodied person who wants to break the cycle of body shame and negativity that surrounds so many of us. We live in a world that constantly pushes us to see ourselves simultaneously as both too much and not enough. The combination of yoga's benefits and body liberation saved my life and changed it forever, and I believe it can do the same for you.

I now live and breathe yoga and body liberation! I never set out to become a yoga teacher, but it happened, and I haven't looked back. I have made it my job to help people find peace and ease in their bodies. I am so grateful to be able to guide folks through figuring out a yoga practice that can develop and deepen over time, eventually becoming an integral part of their lives and a source of healing. Since my first experiences were with yoga teachers who had no idea how to instruct larger bodies, I know exactly what I want to bring into the world. I am here to teach plus-size folks how to make yoga postures work for their bodies and also to spread this knowledge to other yoga teachers so they can better serve their students. I often imagine what it would have been like to have experienced yoga with a knowledgeable teacher way back when. I wasted so many years hating yoga and believing my body was the problem. I don't want people to have the same experiences I did, so I've made it my life's mission to keep that from happening.

I believe we never stop being students, and I love to attend training on a variety of topics and techniques so I can evolve in both my personal practice and as a teacher. Honestly, my life kind of feels like a dream sometimes! I get to do these things that I love and help people at the same time. This book is no exception!

WHAT IS THIS BOOK?

The benefits of yoga are boundless! This is especially true for those who have deeply held shame created by a lifetime of cultural oppression. There is great healing and transformative change to be had for anyone who takes that step to learn and practice yoga. I have lived through this change and believe it can happen for anyone who wants it. A yoga practice can help plus-size folks find deeper self-love and empowerment, as well as freedom, comfort, strength, and mobility in their bodies. This book is a great first step for someone in a larger body looking to access these benefits of yoga. You'll find an overview of common poses, with detailed information about how to use props to create levels of support and ways to find accessible challenges to meet your body where it is. Get creative! Play with different ways to support and move through poses to find a variety of benefits, from strength building to flexibility to reinforcing the mind–body connection. This book is for anyone who wants to explore the practice and philosophy of yoga without body shame or judgment. It is for those who want to connect with themselves in a meaningful way. It's not about weight loss or changing yourself to fit into a beauty standard. Yoga is about empowering yourself and creating meaningful change in how you feel about and feel in your body. Written by and for plus-sized women, I've taken into account our needs and experiences to help you learn how to use props and pose options so you can step into any yoga class and know that you belong there.

HOW CAN THIS BOOK HELP ME?

On these pages, you'll find a wealth of information to guide you through all stages of creating a thriving home yoga practice. You'll learn how to plan for your practice and know that you're prioritizing the safety and comfort of your body. I encourage you to explore ways to physically create a yoga space in your home, set boundaries with yourself and others to prioritize your practice, create yoga sequences that feel complete, and begin thinking of poses in a framework of levels of support and accessible challenges. Become confident and knowledgeable about using props and pose options to give your mind and body what they need, increasing or decreasing support to relax or energize based on how you feel when you step on the mat. I'm including everything I wish I had known as a yoga newbie! Let me help you learn about yoga in a way that is body-positive, fat-friendly, and nonjudgmental. I want to use all the experience I have as a fat yoga practitioner to guide you through the often intimidating world of yoga! I understand the specific needs of a plus-sized body and can't wait to teach you what I know.

I'm so excited to have created this book as a resource for plus-sized folks, featuring photos of actual plus-size bodies! Yoga poses look different on everyone, and this is especially true as bodies get larger. There is often a temptation to try to make your body and pose look like someone else's, which can lead to misalignment and injury over time. Simply put, plus-sized bodies look different in poses than thin bodies. If you are comparing your shape to another's shape, there is great potential for injury and body shame. The photos in this book are for us! They are an incredible tool to help you see what the postures can look like on a variety of larger bodies. They are not only beautiful to see but also help show all the ways props can be used to create levels of support and accessible challenges for each pose we cover. There are multiple options for every pose discussed in this book. I am beyond happy for you to see yourself represented here and learn how to make the yoga poses work for you!

I also can't wait to explore the ever-increasing world of yoga props with you. Companies continually innovate and create new yoga props to add support, challenge, and fun to your practice. Props have become a passion of mine, and I think you'll love them too. We'll dig into which props are useful and even how to make some for yourself. Yoga doesn't have to be expensive! Yoga is for all of us!

Maybe you've tried attending a yoga class before and felt invisible or overly highlighted or simply felt that you didn't belong there. Or perhaps you've wanted to learn more about yoga, but you felt overwhelmed at all the different styles and choices of classes. I get it! I have been through the wringer with yoga, but I came out the other side and have so much to share with you. My greatest hope for anyone reading this book is to see themselves reflected here. I hope you find inspiration and motivation to give yoga a try, especially if you've come to think of the practice as being something that's just not for you. Yoga is so much more than a series of poses and shapes you make with your body. It is a connection between your mind and body that can open you up to self-love and a self-care practice that will stay with you for the rest of your life. Do I sound like a fanatic? I only say these things because my life changed forever when I allowed myself to try again—to be open to this practice we call yoga. I hope that, as you hold this book in your hands, you say yes and start a lifelong relationship with your body and mind that is yours alone to nurture and cherish.

ACKNOWLEDGMENTS

Thank you:

To Richard, who is quite simply my favorite human.

To my family for their unwavering support and cheerleading.

To Natalie, for agreeing to model for this book's photos and for being my friend. I'm honored to be in your life.

To my teachers who changed my life and touched my heart. Abby Lentz and Anna Guest-Jelley, y'all made yoga a possibility for me when I didn't believe.

To Michelle Maloney and the wonderful staff at Human Kinetics. Thank you so much for the opportunity to write this book and help other fat folks access the power of yoga.

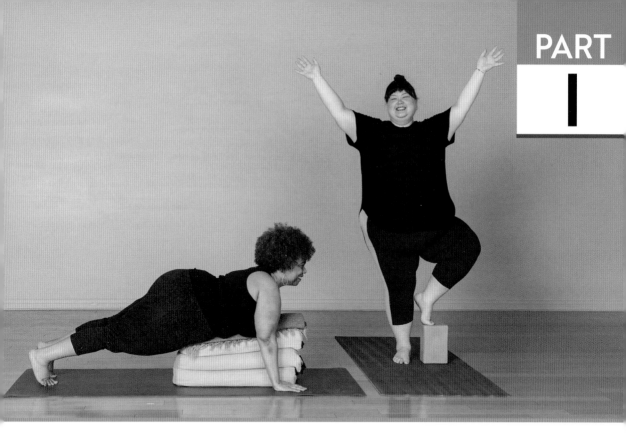

Set for Success

CHAPTER 1

START WITH CONFIDENCE!

The world of yoga can be intimidating for anyone new to it, but it is especially so for those in larger bodies. If you're feeling anxious about beginning your yoga practice, I don't blame you! As a plus-size person who had a rough introduction to yoga (go read the preface if you haven't already), I have learned from the many mistakes that others and I made. I feel very confident in my assertion that many things can go wrong when anyone, much less a larger-bodied person, takes the leap to explore yoga. This is not to scare or convince you that yoga isn't for you. In fact, it's the opposite! Having been through the wringer with my introduction to yoga, I feel particularly qualified to help you navigate this journey with confidence and support. My journey has taught me that not only is yoga for plus-size folks, it is also a strong foundation on which we can build a positive relationship with ourselves.

Let me get this party started with a promise. I will tell you the hard truths about what I wish I had known when I began yoga. I'll give you the information you need to turn a negative situation into a positive one, an empowering step in your journey. The tips I suggest are sometimes difficult to implement, but I've learned that they make all the difference. It can be challenging to change behaviors you've known your whole life; believe me when I say that I get it. Learning to advocate for myself and create a positive community of supportive people has been the ultimate test of my dedication to self-care and body liberation. My goal throughout this book is to help you become empowered to know how to make yoga work for you and confident enough to handle the variety of circumstances you might find yourself in. There were times when I didn't communicate what I needed to teachers and staff in yoga spaces, and I wish I had known how to do that or even that it was an option. This skill and other helpful tips outlined in this chapter are things I didn't know or fully understand when I began my yoga journey. Being unknowledgeable made a difference in my early yoga experiences, but it doesn't have to be that way for you! My job is to make sure you're more enlightened than I was so you can start your yoga journey with strength and confidence in yourself!

This chapter is the beginning of your preparation, and so it is incredibly important because it sets the tone for your personal practice. I know the temptation to skip ahead to the poses and sequences is high, but stick it out and you'll be stronger for it! The tips here will help prepare you for a fun, empowered, and safe exploration of yoga. Some are general tips that are appropriate for anyone exploring yoga, and some are specifically for plus-size practitioners. Regardless, all the information here will be helpful for you as you begin to find your place within the world of yoga. Whether you plan on attending in-person classes in your town, streaming practices from the comfort of your home, or simply following along with the sequences in this book, the information here will help you be your best advocate for a safe and empowered yoga practice!

GENERAL TIPS FOR ANYONE EXPLORING YOGA

It's totally natural to experience anxiety when learning something new, and I am willing to bet pretty much every yoga newbie felt the same way during her introduction to yoga. I sure did! Luckily for us, this feeling is so common that there are tons of resources out there to help you prepare. There are lots of online articles and blogs, magazine features, and studio welcome pages that speak to the beginner yogi's questions and anxieties about trying yoga. A quick search can teach you everything from snacks before class that won't upset your stomach to basic yoga gear to tips on how to find a yoga studio that fits your needs and lifestyle. These types of resources can be helpful, and I encourage you to read and soak up everything you can about your new practice. That kind of research was helpful for me, but like many things in life, my most impactful lessons came from real-life experience. I dove headfirst into yoga without knowing much, and honestly, I wish I hadn't. A little more information would have helped me make smarter choices and feel more competent as I tried studios and classes. I've curated the recommendations in this chapter based on these lessons. Everything outlined here is on my list of "What I wish I had heard before I hit the mat the first time."

> *I have been a seeker and I still am, but I stopped asking the books and the stars. I started listening to the teaching of my Soul.*
>
> Rumi

For a newcomer, deciphering the differences between styles of yoga is incredibly important. In the beginning, I didn't understand that I could be selective about the style of yoga and the type of classes I attended. I didn't fully understand that I could choose classes that fit my goals and lifestyle, and that yoga styles were so varied and nuanced. I looked around and saw mostly one or two types of classes, and so those were the types I thought I should like. At first, I tried to make myself fit into the type of yoga that I saw in most of the local studios, and I was miserable! It took me a while, but I finally figured out that finding my footing in the realm of yoga was a lot easier when I honored my needs. Trying to force yourself to like a style of yoga that's just not for you will not give you the benefits you need. Please don't waste your time like I did!

Second to finding the right yoga style and class type, I think that maintaining a sense of humor about the process is very important. You will likely encounter experiences and classes that push you out of your comfort zone. You might be late to class, trip over your own feet, and, yes, you'll probably fart in class at some point! The best way to deal with these and other awkward situations is to keep your sense of humor at the forefront and try not to take yourself too seriously. Add to this list the important task of meeting your body where it is. This is easy to say and harder to do in practice, but starting out in a mindful way can save you a lot of heartache and frustration. Adjust your expectations, and be as kind to yourself as you would be to your best friend.

Find the Type of Yoga Class That's Right for You

I wish you could have seen me, young and just getting into yoga, in a steaming-hot room trying to keep up with experienced yogis. I must have radiated unhappiness from every part of me! The sad part is that I went back, time and again, even though I hated the class. I felt like I had to keep going back, despite the fact that these classes left me feeling unseen, unteachable, and unhappy with my body. I tried hot yoga, power yoga, kundalini yoga, ashtanga yoga, and lots of other classes that never felt right for me. I didn't leave feeling blissed out like so many other students did. I walked out of these studios feeling sad, angry, embarrassed, and confused. I internalized every bad experience and every unpleasant class until I was convinced yoga just wasn't for people like me. It took a long time to figure out that I thrive in gentle hatha classes with options to create accessible challenges for myself, and that I love restorative yoga and meditation. Learning to leave behind the classes that weren't right for me changed my view on yoga permanently. Empowering myself to say "no" completely reset my mindset about what I deserve to do and feel in my life, and especially in terms of health and fitness.

Now I know what I like, what my body responds to, and that if I don't like a class, it's not my body's fault for not being good enough. This new perspective has opened a world of possibilities for me, and I hope it will do the same for you. In my life, this empowerment means that I give myself permission to use props in class, not to "fix the problem" of my body, but to make the pose work for my body and what it needs. I love experimenting with the gentle support of a chair class, the slow deep stretch of a yin class, or the peace of a restorative class. I encourage you to try different types of classes, but also give yourself permission to not go back if it doesn't feel right. You'll know if you liked a type of class, and there's no need to punish yourself by attempting to force a love for something that doesn't light you up. Just because something is popular doesn't mean you have to like it or that it's right for you. I know that sounds simple, but I find that many of my students have fallen into the same trap I did. We tried to make ourselves enjoy the forms of yoga that are marketed as weight loss or body shaping because we thought that was what we deserved for being bigger. We were trying to punish ourselves for our size. I hope that you are kind and compassionate with yourself and investigate the classes that feel good and fill you with peace, confidence, and ease in your body. You might find that you love intense classes that leave you sweaty and with muscles that feel like limp noodles. Or you may discover a love for classes with dimly lit rooms and candlelight. Just make sure you love a class because it makes you feel great, not because you think it's where you're supposed to be.

Hatha yoga spawned the Iyengar, ashtanga, and vinyasa styles of yoga we see practiced today. While these are styles of yoga, many classes offered will be named after them. You may not see a power vinyasa class. Instead, the class may simply be called vinyasa or flow yoga. Be prepared to see a wide variety of class names; a studio tends to have its own way of phrasing and naming classes. If you understand the differences between the yoga styles, you should be able to decipher what kind of class is being offered.

Here are brief explanations of some of the types of classes you might find at your local studio, online, and in this book. I hope this helps you begin to learn about the options available and gives you an idea of the type of classes you might gravitate toward.

Hatha

This style of yoga is rooted in the combination of physical postures (asana) and breath work (pranayama). While other styles of yoga were created based on hatha, it remains one of the most practiced styles. Generally, a hatha class will be a relatively gentle class, with a more relaxed feeling and longer hold times for poses. General hatha classes are typically good for beginners because the slower pace, use of props, and attention to alignment are great for learning basic postures.

Iyengar

Often compared closely to the original hatha style, Iyengar is another yoga form that values alignment and the use of props. Students healing from injury are typically referred to Iyengar classes due to the meticulous focus on proper alignment and liberal use of support in postures.

Ashtanga

Classes in this style are dynamic, energizing, and can demand a lot from students. Sticking with a set sequence each time, ashtanga classes ask students to move from one posture to the next without stopping. This style is typically physically challenging and fast-paced.

Vinyasa

These classes are known for their fluid movement and creative sequencing, and they are often physically demanding. Vinyasa classes are focused on linking movement with breath, and students flow from one pose directly into the next. However, not all vinyasa classes are so fast-paced, and slow-flow classes are becoming more popular with practitioners who want a slower-moving sequence.

Chair Yoga

In chair yoga, classes are taught either exclusively with, or complemented by, a chair and other props. Not just for older folks or those recovering from injury, chair classes are a great way to find support in poses and experience them in new and interesting ways. Chair classes are often, but not always, gentle and slow moving. However, there are plenty of ways to incorporate chairs into your practice and find many accessible challenges.

Power Yoga

Sometimes confused for ashtanga classes, power yoga classes are fitness-focused and prioritize energetic, physically demanding sequences. Like ashtanga yoga, power yoga classes move quickly, and practitioners do not stay in any one pose for a long time. However, the differences between the two types of classes are easily seen in the sequencing. While ashtanga repeats the same sequence each time, power yoga classes offer a mix of postures in each class. Some studios offer heated rooms for power yoga, but some are cooler-temperature classes. Be sure to check ahead of time so you know what kind of class it is!

Hot Yoga

Different styles of yoga are offered under the umbrella of hot yoga. Most people think of Bikram yoga, a type of class composed of a specific sequence of poses taught in a very hot room. While the Bikram name is the most commonly known when it comes to hot yoga, it's not the only kind! Studios offer various types of hot yoga classes with temperatures from 80 to 105 degrees Fahrenheit (27 to 41 degrees Celsius), many different sequences, longer or shorter postural holds, and teaching philosophies that differ greatly.

Beginner Yoga

Beginner classes are offered everywhere and in every style of yoga. They are a great place to start your yoga journey, and many folks continue to take these classes for years. Beginner classes aren't just for newbie yogis! The strong focus on the basics of alignment, breath work, and meditation are important for all practitioners of yoga. Even if you eventually move on to other types of classes, coming back occasionally to take beginner classes is a smart practice.

Yin Yoga

Deceptively simple and slow, yin classes offer in-depth attention to alignment, long holds in each posture, and a mindfulness practice that keeps you present in your body. The poses and longer hold lengths allow your body to stretch not only the muscles but also the connective tissue and fascia, leading to deeper impact.

Restorative Yoga

Restorative yoga provides a relaxing and healing class that uses props to support the body so you can truly release tension. Restorative classes are a great way to find some ease in your day, calm your nervous system, be present in your body without outside distractions, and focus on breathing exercises to cultivate certain sensations or energy in your body. Slow, quiet, and nurturing, restorative classes give you space to be introspective and gently stretch and rest.

Prenatal Yoga

Prenatal yoga consists of gentle yoga classes designed specifically to ease common pains related to pregnancy, foster the relationship between you and your baby, reduce your stress, and improve sleep. Instructors will have completed prenatal yoga training that teaches them the best poses to help a host of needs specific to pregnant people.

Aerial Yoga

Aerial yoga pairs common yoga poses with elements of acrobatic fitness that require suspended silk hammocks to lift you into the air. Beginner classes focus on familiarizing students with the silks and trying basic aerial moves. More advanced classes bring a higher level of difficulty and combine a series of acrobatic moves into a vinyasa-style sequence both on and off the floor.

There are so many styles of classes to try, and I encourage you to mix it up! I definitely fell into the trap of thinking that power yoga, or any other very athletic and gymnastic yoga classes, were what I should be taking and didn't fully give other classes a chance. I believed that my job as a yoga newbie was to fall in line with whatever the predominant yoga offerings were, regardless of whether I enjoyed them or was benefiting from them. This is a lesson I can't stress enough to you. *Find the yoga that speaks to you, not the yoga you think you're supposed to like.* The types of classes listed here and so many more are available to you in person and online. It can be really fun to explore them to see what fits your body and lifestyle best.

It can also be uncomfortable, awkward, and traumatic. Remember when I told you I'd tell you the truth, even if it's not the easiest? When, or if, you feel ready to try out a new type of class, do your research. What kind of studio is offering it? Does it seem to focus on weight loss or changing your body? Does the marketing language make you feel uncomfortable? What kind of images do you find on the studio's social media? Look for places that encourage you to explore how it feels to practice in their style rather than on what you look like. Gaining strength, losing weight, and becoming flexible are all things that *might* happen once you begin your yoga practice. They also might not. Find the yoga that makes you feel energized, calm, easy in your body, or connected with your inner self. Find the yoga that works for your body and your specific needs. Embrace your natural curiosity, and try classes if they sound exciting or interesting. Take a safe risk! Aerial yoga? Why not? Cat yoga? Yes please! Just remember that you are the boss when it comes to your body. Ultimately, the decision of which type of classes to take is up to you, and there's nothing you need to prioritize over your safety, comfort, and experience.

Your Sense of Humor Can Save You

There are lots of times in yoga when it's easy to become discouraged, embarrassed, or jealous of situations and other people. This is especially true for new students of yoga. In the beginning, there is often a tendency to focus on your perceived faults. It's human nature to notice your weakness, inflexibility, and racing mind, and to compare it to the practiced postures and mindfulness of other students. Some of the best tools you have in your self-care toolbox are humor and patience, and they often work hand in hand! Finding the humor in situations when you might otherwise be tempted to feel shame or embarrassment is a wonderful way of practicing self-care. We are all new at something at one time or another, and very few come to yoga already flexible, balanced, and deeply mindful. Despite knowing this, we tend to be unkind to ourselves and foster unreasonable expectations. We are quick to find fault with ourselves and often approach our behavior or actions with much less kindness and compassion than we show others. We would never expect these criticisms from other folks, yet we are cruel taskmasters with ourselves.

Remind yourself that even the most flexible and centered yogis began their journeys at some point. If you fall asleep in savasana, or deep-relaxation pose, smile at your sleepiness! If you fall over in a balance pose, giggle! If you pass gas in class, laugh it off! We all break wind in class at some point, even the teachers! The kindest thing you can do for yourself is to smile, laugh it off, and move on.

Channeling your most patient and lighthearted self and reminding your inner critic that you're doing your best are difficult and rewarding practices. So much of yoga is an exploration of our bodies, sensations, experiences, and perspectives about life in general. Sometimes exploration leads to awkward moments, and sometimes it leads to epiphanies—and the two are not mutually exclusive! Keep your sense of humor and ride the waves of emotion. This is yoga. Something embarrasses you? Practice svadhyaya, or self-inquiry, and ask why you're feeling that way and what it would mean to let go of your embarrassment. A yoga practice can bring up a lot of different kinds of emotions, and it's not uncommon for practitioners to feel anger, hurt, and happiness or to cry in class. You may experience discomfort in your body or mind, find yourself with heightened emotions seemingly out of nowhere, or need to stop your practice and rest for the remainder of class. All these experiences are part of yoga, and the kindest thing you can do for yourself is to approach your practice with humor, self-compassion, and patience.

Meet Your Body Where It Is

I have to tell you, I am the queen of letting expectations get the best of me. It's not something I like about myself, but I accept that it's true, and I'm working on it. I've been working on it for a long time! This, and so many of the lessons I've learned through yoga, is a lifelong practice of vulnerability and compassion. It's human nature to be highly critical of ourselves and kind to others. We set grand expectations for ourselves, only to be let down when our real experiences don't stack up. I just want to remind you how unkind that is! Do yourself a favor and don't worry about how flexible or strong you think you should be. Release expectations of perfectly Zen meditation and open yourself up to being exactly where you are. It's a common tendency to think we should be faster, stronger, smarter, and further along in our individual journeys than we are. This mindset is damaging, unfair, and simply unhelpful. Instead, try being open to seeing where your body and mind truly are however flexible, strong, and meditative you find yourself. Let that be your starting point. Meet yourself exactly where you are, not where you think you should be.

> *Yoga begins right where I am, not where I was yesterday or where I long to be.*
>
> Linda Sparrowe

Our bodies are different every day, and the pose you struggled with last week might feel rooted and strong today. Or not! You have the rest of your life to gain flexibility, strength, and a mindful presence. True self-care is about meeting yourself where you are, releasing expectations, and opening yourself

Start With Confidence! ▪ 11

to the present. Welcome! It might be messier here, but at least it's real. Part of doing the work of yoga is allowing yourself to find and stay in that messy space. Yoga asks you to identify what your body needs in each moment and to let those needs guide your practice.

Sometimes our bodies are energetic and craving a movement practice that brings our focus to muscles and breath in a way that warms us and emphasizes building heat. On these days, a faster-paced sequence with lots of movement could be the perfect practice. Other days, our bodies and minds let us know that minimal movement, softness, and restoration are what we need. Choosing a meditation practice with gentle breath work and a nice, long savasana might be the best course of action here. By getting present in our bodies and asking what they need, we are creating a personal culture of kindness and self-care. After all, what good is a yoga practice if it's the means of suffering and punishment? You don't owe anyone a sweaty power yoga practice! You don't owe anyone a guided meditation! You only owe yourself compassion and permission to be exactly as you are, to move in whatever ways feel best.

TIPS FOR PLUS-SIZE YOGIS, LEARNED THE HARD WAY

Alright y'all, here we go! This is where I really dig into the tips that apply to those of us in larger bodies. These pieces of wisdom, learned through personal experience, can help you build a stronger yoga practice and grow as a person. I've included recommendations that have truly served me the most as a plus-size practitioner of yoga. Of course, while any tips you find for newbie yogis are helpful, there are some things that solely apply to folks like us. Living in larger bodies comes with benefits and challenges that other people can't know because it's outside of their experience. They don't know because they've never had to know, but I'm in this with you and have been where you are! I'm committed and so happy to be able to help you navigate the areas that can be challenging for plus-size people. I have been through all of this and more! My introduction to yoga was traumatic, and the memories and feelings have informed the way I teach and my philosophy about yoga. My goal here is to give you the information to have a happier, smoother, easier, and more positive introduction to yoga. I know that it can feel like yoga isn't for those of us in bigger bodies, but it is! Yoga is for every body!

One of the pieces of wisdom I've learned along the way from my amazing yoga teachers, Anna Guest-Jelley of Curvy Yoga and Abby Lentz of HeavyWeight Yoga, is that *our bodies are not a problem to be solved*. We come to yoga, not to change them, but to change the way we think about them. Yoga can help us know ourselves and find a deeper connection to our bodies we may have never had before. This was certainly true for me, and I hope that it will be true for you.

Your body is not a problem to be solved.

The tips that follow were learned the hard way, through situations I hope you'll never experience. I've compiled information that I wish I'd known as I explored yoga for the first time. Learn from my mistakes and spare yourself the heartache and injury!

The Yoga Industry Is Behind the Times

The body-positivity movement has gained a lot of traction in the United States and continues to create meaningful change in many areas of life. We larger-bodied folks have more support and visibility than ever before. Even as few as five years ago, there was a distinct difference in the quantity and quality of access to wellness and fitness spaces. There is amazing advocacy work being done by plus-size activists around the globe! Unfortunately, the world of yoga is a little behind. While a few bigger-bodied yoga practitioners and teachers have gained a following and are able to spread their messages of equality and accessibility, changes are slow to come to yoga studios, trainings, and teachers.

The business of yoga is booming, and studios are producing yoga instructors in large numbers, but without much experience in teaching plus-size students. These teachers are attending trainings that do not spend much, or any, time on how to work with *all* kinds of bodies or even how to integrate props seamlessly into their classes. Compounding the problem is the societal focus on dieting and the internalized weight stigma that flourishes in many yoga spaces. Whether consciously or not, many yoga teachers create classes rooted in diet culture and body shaming. I've personally experienced this in almost every studio class I've ever taken! There are constant mentions of poses that will create fat loss, weight changes, and targeted body shrinking. I've had teachers ask me how much weight I'd like to lose before they bother to ask my name. I've seen teachers announce how many calories were burned during class, reading off their smart watches and instructing us to keep our dinners light so we don't ruin our progress. One teacher put her hand on my belly and rattled off a number of poses I could practice daily to get rid of it. Unfortunately, I have many more examples of behavior like this, but I'll spare you the negativity.

This weight stigma is often carried throughout every part of American yoga culture, and it starts in the teacher trainings. This negative bias is slowly changing, but the unpleasant fact is that people in larger bodies need to be prepared every time we go to a new studio. Until the standard of behavior changes and teacher trainings add accessibility education to their curriculum, we need to be ready for the fact that we might walk into a class and have a teacher who is both not ready to teach us safely and also not inclined to do so respectfully.

Inexperienced Teachers Might Make Things Weird

The lack of training described previously can lead to problems when students in larger bodies show up to class. Inexperienced teachers might be both excited to teach them and also completely unprepared to do so. When I've taken class from a teacher who has no idea what to do with my body, there are typically two reactions to my presence that occur. The first is when the teacher will enthusiastically greet me and then proceed to overly highlight me throughout the duration of class. This can include, but is not limited to, asking the rest of class to watch me in a pose, calling attention to my alignment, complimenting my flexibility or strength, asking me to demo a posture for the class, or praising me much more than anyone in the class. I believe this comes from a good place and the teacher just wants me to feel welcomed and supported. Unfortunately, this behavior simply succeeds in singling me out and making me (and the other students) feel uncomfortable. The second reaction is the exact opposite, which means the teacher doesn't make any effort to greet me, ask if I have any injuries, offer postural cues, or otherwise interact with me in any way. Both behaviors lead to me feeling awkward, uncomfortable, and ready to leave and never return!

Yoga teachers learn about alignment and teaching techniques from models and each other during teacher training. Most folks taking teacher trainings are straight sized, or what many would describe as thin. If yoga teachers are learning about alignment with only straight-size examples, then they are not learning how to teach plus-size students. Larger bodies can look different than smaller bodies when holding yoga postures. Larger bodies may require different options to get proper alignment and the intended benefit of poses. Many teachers are simply unequipped to help plus-size students get the benefits of yoga. Don't get me wrong, I think straight-size yoga instructors can be wonderful teachers for plus-size folks if they get the training they need! I don't think they set out to bring body shame to their classes, but sometimes their training lets them down.

During class, teachers will cue you to come into poses and give you information about proper alignment, including where you might feel stretching or which muscles might be working, etc. Since plus-size bodies can look very different in yoga poses than their straight-sized counterparts, there is the possibility that an inexperienced teacher might give you misguided alignment corrections that could cause harm. A yoga teacher with little experience working with larger bodies might look at your body, see that it looks different than other folks in the room, think misalignment is to blame, and then have you adjust your position through verbal cues or hands-on physical adjustment. This can be dangerous if you're actually already in proper alignment. The danger might be as simple as making you second-guess yourself, leading you to doubt your own knowledge of your body. Or the danger could be physical, with repeated misalignment mistakes causing injury over time. This is why it's so important for us to learn how alignment in supposed to *feel* and to not focus on how a pose looks.

Learning what proper alignment feels like in your body will empower you to know that you are getting the benefits of each pose, even when your teacher might think you are out of alignment. It can be helpful to tell your teacher what you're feeling in your body so she can understand that you are actually in the correct alignment and getting what you need out of the pose. Every time you teach your yoga instructor how alignment can look in a larger body, she is better equipped to teach plus-size students in the future! Every time you trust yourself and maintain boundaries, you are helping to create a change in our culture and supporting the plus-size yogis who come after you.

This book will help prepare you for situations like these, learning great options for commonly taught poses that will keep you safely supported and confident in any yoga class. If you know how to use props to make the yoga poses work for you, you can take that knowledge anywhere and turn any mediocre class into a great practice! It's empowering to know how to support your body, especially when your teacher doesn't know how to properly teach you. The information in this book is a great start for learning how to support yourself and find accessible challenges, no matter what kind of class or teacher you find yourself matched with.

Classes May Turn Out to Be Different Than You Thought

You might walk into a new class with all the confidence in the world and quickly discover it's not what you expected. Sometimes classes turn out to be a different style of yoga than you thought they would be. Or you'll find that the teacher has a teaching style that doesn't fit your needs. Or maybe there's some other reason that you don't feel comfortable in a specific class. It may be that the sequence is moving faster than you had anticipated or that the teacher isn't using any props in class. You may need to advocate for yourself by bringing as many props as you'd like to your mat. Or it might be that resting briefly or until class is over is the right thing for you that day.

Also, remember that you don't have to stick it out! Your job is to decide if you want to stay for the rest of class or if the best thing you could do for yourself is leave. There are a ton of reasons why you might decide to leave a class once it's begun, and, honestly, it doesn't matter what your particular reason is. You never have to stay in a class that doesn't feel good to you. Don't worry about hurting the teacher's feelings or being disruptive. Your biggest priority is protecting yourself! This is self-care. If you want to explain to the instructor, send an email or other communication after you leave. Don't pull the instructor's attention away from teaching to explain in the moment why you're leaving.

You Are the Boss of Your Body

As you deepen your yoga practice, you will learn what feels safe, what works for you, and how proper alignment feels in your body in a range of poses. Once you know these things, it's only a matter of claiming your power and advocating for yourself. If a class, teacher, pose, or an instruction isn't right for you and you're not feeling safe or respected, you can leave, stop, or do something else! You don't have to stay for a whole class if you don't feel safe or respected. You are the only one who gets to decide if you receive hands-on adjustment, if an alignment cue is correct for your body, and whether you want to go deeper or push harder with a particular pose. You can decide that a conversation about weight loss or dieting isn't for you. As the boss of your body, you decide what your boundaries are regarding every aspect of class, social interactions with teachers and students, and the yoga communities you become part of. Never be afraid to put yourself and your safety first! Setting boundaries is a tool in your self-care toolbox that can keep you safe in any circumstance.

The importance of body autonomy should never be underestimated! Body autonomy is the right of each person to decide what happens with her body at all times. Often discussed in terms of consent, there are many situations in which body autonomy comes into play in yoga spaces. Teachers wanting to correct my alignment have touched me or given me hugs and diet advice—all without my consent. I have had teachers and studio owners discuss my body's perceived flaws in front of me but while speaking to each other as if I weren't there. I have been offered diet tips, weight loss advice, clothing style advice, and every type of unsolicited human interaction. These behaviors frequently happen to plus-size people because our culture generally does not value our bodily autonomy. This is where you have to step up and be an advocate for yourself. Creating and maintaining boundaries is one of the best ways to create a culture of consent and respect around your body. When you show people that you know your body and will make your own choices, it teaches them how to treat you. This has been a long-term practice for me, with many ups and downs. I have experienced the power of showing others how I want to be treated! It really does make a difference for you and for the rest of our community.

Comparing Yourself to Others Only Leads to Problems

One of the most helpful things I've learned during my years of yoga practice is that comparing myself to other people is neither healthy nor helpful. I suppose this is a lesson that's true for all parts of life, but I find it especially helpful in yoga spaces. It's very easy to look at magazines, TV, online yoga spaces, and in-person classes and see folks in poses that seem glamorous and impressive. These seem to be the only kind of poses that get offered up for our consumption, and the intent is to make us want to be like these "flawless" yogis. Yoga is often presented to us as an aspirational practice that encourages us to strive to look and act like the famous yoga teachers and influencers. This is dangerous territory! Comparing ourselves to these people and trying to be like them isn't fair to us or to them. This kind of mindset can lead to negative self-image, mistrust of your body and mind, and an unhealthy preoccupation with feeling that you're not where you should be.

Comparison is the thief of joy.

Theodore Roosevelt

Some people are naturally flexible, strong, or quicker to learn new skills than others. What may look like an amazing feat of yoga asana might be an easy pose to the person you're watching. We all have our own unique skills and talents, and what is easy for some is potentially impossible for others. There are certain poses, found in every yoga magazine or social media account, that are impressive to see and absolutely the product of a body that has the right ratio of limb lengths to flexibility to pull the poses off. There are common poses that some of us will never be able to achieve without props because the length of our arms and legs just won't get us there. And there's nothing wrong with that! There's nothing wrong with using props to make the pose work for your body. Your version of a pose doesn't need to look like anyone else's version. Yoga is not a competition.

Furthermore, there's no rule that says your yoga practice needs to have the same goals as anyone else's practice. Instead of thinking of yoga as a practice to get your body to be like someone else's, think about what you truly want from yoga. For me, yoga is a practice that keeps me connected to my body so that I don't become disconnected from myself again. Yoga helps me to be present and focused on keeping the mind–body connection alive and vibrant. My yoga practice helps me move in ways that feel good, find greater strength and flexibility, and connect with myself and others in more meaningful ways. If your goal for your yoga practice is to become connected with yourself, that's great! If your goal is to learn how to push your body and find your greatest strength and focus, wonderful! However, if you're comparing yourself and your body to others as a way to measure progress, I would warn you to rethink your perspective for your own good. I truly believe that nothing good comes from comparing yourself to other people.

A flower does not think of competing to the flower next to it. It just blooms.

Zen Shin Meditation (Ogui)

Not only is comparing yourself to others a potentially harmful way to think, but it simply isn't fair. When you watch someone engage in her yoga practice, all you can see is what is visible to your eyes. You can't see how long she worked on that pose, the natural flexibility or strength she started with, the number of times she tried and failed to master that pose, or anything else beyond what is right in front of you. It's unfair to yourself to compare your body and mind to anyone else's. You may be watching someone who has practiced a pose for years. You may be watching someone who spent her childhood learning gymnastics. Or you may be watching someone with a ton of natural aptitude for physical asana. Judging yourself against another isn't fair to you, and it's also not fair to her. You probably know what it feels like to have someone look at you and judge your body and skills. I know that, for me, it feels terrible. It's unfair to bring our comparison and judgment to an unwilling outsider who is simply enjoying her personal yoga practice.

Comparing yourself to another yoga student is also potentially dangerous. These comparisons often lead to pushing yourself harder than what is safe and attempting poses that your body or mind isn't ready for. When you see folks with different body types in the same pose as you, there may be differences in what you see. Different kinds of bodies look different in poses all the time! It's not bad, it's just different. Trust yourself to know that you're feeling the benefit of the pose and that you're in the correct alignment. Don't worry about the shapes someone else is making—trust yourself. Forcing yourself into misalignment just to make yourself look like other people is dangerous and can lead to injury. We're all moving through the world together, but on different paths. Stay on your path with your own timeline. Your yoga practice may look very different from mine, and that's okay! Yoga thrives on difference and diversity!

Trust in Yourself Is the Ultimate Yoga Resource

I came to the world of yoga with a lifetime of disconnection, mistrust, and unease in my body. I didn't feel particularly confident about anything regarding my body, much less about what it needed, how it felt, or what it could do. I say this because some of you may be in a similar situation. I find that it's common for folks to come to yoga as a step in their journey to self-love, and then struggle with trusting their own feelings and intuition. It's not easy to trust yourself when you've spent your life being told your body, behaviors, and desires are wrong. If this feels true for you, take heart! Learning to trust yourself gets easier as you practice, and yoga offers many chances to do just that.

Your yoga practice will ask you to take safe risks, whether physically or mentally. Each time you take on one of these risks and come out stronger, you will trust yourself more! Whether it's a balance pose that requires you to trust the strength of your body, or pranayama (breath work) that asks you to breathe in new ways that may be uncomfortable at first, a huge part of yoga is developing trust in yourself as the expert on your body. You are the only one who can feel what is happening inside, and, therefore, you are the world's foremost expert on yourself! Practice trusting yourself just as you will practice meditation techniques and yoga postures. This trust will help you in many ways, including protecting yourself from misguided outside influences and the human desire to compare ourselves with others.

CONCLUSION

All these recommendations from me can be boiled down into a few words: Be kind to yourself and trust your body. Kindness is important when it comes to learning any new skill, especially when it involves your body and your relationship with your body. The world of yoga can be overwhelming and intimidating, with lots of outside emphasis on expensive leggings and gymnastic poses. The kindest thing you can do for yourself is to let those outside influences fall away and focus on finding what feels best in your body and mind. This is truly self-kindness at its core. Asking your body what it needs and finding ways to honor those needs is self-care that will bolster you through the difficult times in life.

Trusting yourself may feel incredibly challenging at first, especially if you're like me and have spent a large portion of your life not trusting your desires and thoughts. Working on finding that trust with your mind and body will help you build the confidence to become a strong self-advocate in classes and relationships with yoga teachers and other yogis. Some of the most empowering moments have been when I advocated for myself in class and taught my yoga teachers about working with larger-bodied students. This is not to say that you shouldn't trust or listen to yoga teachers! They are trained in the science and art of teaching yoga and are amazing resources for you to learn from. What I want you to take away from this chapter is that you are ultimately the one in charge of your body, and you know it best. Your mental and physical well-being are your priorities, and focusing on them will never steer you wrong. Learning to advocate for yourself will strengthen your yoga practice and contribute to your continued journey toward self-love and self-care.

CHAPTER 2

GET YOUR GEAR

I don't know about you, but when I start a new hobby or movement form, I get excited to explore all the materials or gear that I think I'll need. Sometimes I go a little overboard and end up spending a ton of money on stuff I really don't need. Does this sound familiar? This chapter is here to help you learn about what yoga gear is out there and how much of it you actually need. I'm going to talk to you about what to look for in quality clothing and props, how these tools can help your practice be safer and more enjoyable, and how to make your own version of some of them or find household swaps. If you like DIYing, you're in luck!

First though, I want to talk to you about yoga props in general. If you're like me when I first started yoga, you may have the idea that props are for those who are weak or who just can't do the poses correctly without them. I get it! When I first began practicing yoga, I believed that using props was a weakness and that I didn't need them. I wasted so much time suffering through classes and actually ended up injuring myself because I refused to use any props! I felt like I needed to prove something to other people and to myself, and that ego-driven decision led me to injuries that still pop up to this day. I was so stuck in thinking that I needed to show other people that bigger-bodied folks could do yoga just like they could, that we were just as good and worthy, that I permanently harmed myself. It seems unreal to see that written out, and it's a good reminder of how much it's possible to change. My relationship with props, pose options, and personal challenges has changed dramatically in the years since my first class. While intellectually I know how unnecessary my old way of thinking and behaving was, I completely understand the urge. If you find yourself thinking in this same way, I hope that you learn from my experiences and allow yourself to explore the wonderful world of yoga props and all the benefits they bring. I can't wait to dive into the rest of the chapter and sing the praises of what these props can do!

CHOOSING THE BEST CLOTHING FOR YOUR PRACTICE

Clothing may seem like a frivolous topic, but wearing the right clothing can do wonders to boost your yoga practice. I have bought and tested activewear clothing from numerous plus-size retailers over the years and can confidently say that a bad outfit can ruin your practice! The clothing you choose does much more than make your butt look cute; it not only provides stability, support, and health and safety benefits, but also contributes to your overall sense of confidence. The right clothing can set you up to feel strong, confident, and focused—on your practice, not your pants!

The best yoga clothing items will keep your body comfortable, protected, dry, and will not impede your movement or sight. We all inhabit very different bodies with individual needs, but at our core, we need to feel supported, safe, and comfortable. There are lots of different styles of yoga clothing that practitioners choose to wear, from loose-fitting, pajama-style outfits to the modern yogi's tight-fitting leggings and sports bras. It's up to you to figure out what you feel most comfortable, safe, and supported in. This is your practice and your outfit choice!

Keep in mind what kind of yoga practice or style you will be engaging in. A restorative class and a power yoga class will have very different needs in terms of style and materials. Think through your specific needs before spending money on a new yoga outfit. You may already have exactly what you need! Generally speaking, a gentle class with less movement such as restorative yoga or yin yoga can be done in the widest array of clothing options. Some students may choose to attend these classes in loose-fitting clothing made of natural fibers or even pajamas. Some might choose the tighter-fitting synthetic fabric garments made popular in power yoga and hot yoga classes. In those dynamic power yoga and hot yoga classes, as well as many other types of classes with lots of movement, sweating, and inversions, you will find most students opting for the tight-fitting synthetic material clothing that wicks sweat quickly away and clings to the body to keep movement and sight lines free. Your outfit choice can be very important to your overall enjoyment of a class. Trust me, you haven't lived until you've almost suffocated in an inversion because your face is stuck inside your voluminous cotton T-shirt that's heavy with sweat and hanging down in front of you!

Regardless of the type of class you'll be participating in, the most important criteria for choosing a yoga outfit are whether or not you feel comfortable, supported, and safe! Stability and support are critical for those concerned with keeping their breasts from bouncing or cutting off air supply or sight in certain postures. Being choked by your chest is a problem for a lot of yoga practitioners, plus size or not! Look for materials with compression levels that give you the support you need. Compression in the material can also help reduce muscle fatigue and soreness after a challenging practice.

Choosing a material with sweat-wicking properties can be a great help in keeping your body both safe and healthy. Wicking tops and pants will quickly move sweat away from your body and dry fast to keep you from slipping around on your mat and potentially getting injured. The wicking action will also help to keep your body dry, which can be helpful in preventing yeast infections caused by wearing tight clothing, wet with sweat, for long periods of time. Additionally, bulky or wet seams on clothing can cause chafing on the sensitive skin of your inner thighs, underarms, and belly.

Ultimately, clothing is important for many reasons that affect the happiness, safety, and satisfaction you feel about your yoga practice. Choosing your outfits with care is part of your journey with yoga. While it can be fun to experiment with different styles, colors, materials, and combinations of items, it's understandable if you're feeling trepidation at the thought of finding the right clothing for you. As plus-sized people, we have much less access to activewear, especially high-quality activewear in truly inclusive sizing. I know how challenging it can be to shop for any plus-sized clothing, and yoga clothing is even harder to find. Luckily for us, there are more options now than ever before! While our selection isn't as varied as what is available for straight-sized shoppers, there are great yoga clothes to be found at all price points. It is possible to get the clothing you need, at the price you can pay, to help you feel confident and empowered in your practice!

Where to Look

No matter what your needs and budget are, there are places where you can find activewear to get yourself ready for your practice. I'm excited to talk to you about some of my favorite ways to find yoga clothes, so let's dig in! If you're willing to spend some time searching, you can find anything you need and get a great deal!

My first advice? Start with what you have. Many people are surprised to see that they have all the yoga clothes they need in their closet already! Before you hit the mall, put your wallet away and see what you already have that will work for your needs. Most of us already own joggers, leggings, pajama pants, bike shorts, or other stretchy and comfortable bottoms that will work just fine for most yoga classes. Plus, tank tops, T-shirts, and other activewear tops are great for all sorts of yoga practices. So, head to your closet and do a little shopping from your existing wardrobe. If you don't find everything you need, you can hit the stores, both in-person and online.

If you're ready to start shopping at stores, please allow me to suggest starting at your local thrift or consignment stores. I don't always find a ton in my size, but I have scored big often enough for me to recommend this to you! While the plus-size section of these stores tends to be much smaller than the straight-sized area, there are awesome deals to be found if you get lucky. Be sure to check if there is a separate activewear section for plus sizes so you don't miss out. Sometimes all plus-sized clothing is together and sometimes it's separated, so thrift and consignment shopping can take extra effort. It's worth it when you find a sweet deal on otherwise expensive clothes you wouldn't have been able to afford. If you strike out, or thrifting isn't for you, it's time to move on to the brick-and-mortar stores in your area.

If you're a frequent shopper, you'll probably have a good idea of the stores in your town that have sizes and prices that work for you. If not, it would be helpful to do a little online research to make sure whichever stores you decide to visit have clothing in your size in the store.

Unfortunately, some stores don't choose to stock their larger sizes in their stores. It's such a bummer to drive all the way to a store and have your excitement dashed when you realize there's nothing there for you to try on. Ask me how I know! If you're confident that the store has your size there to try on, head on over and check it out. You may already have a good idea of what their activewear is like, but if you don't, it's important to give yourself a good chunk of time to look it over and try things on! Don't be afraid to ask an employee questions about the items you're interested in. If the tags and signage don't say, ask about the material's benefits, the fit, other size options, etc. This may sound basic to some of you, but plenty of us have spent a lot of years feeling unworthy or scared of asking for help or more information. So, here's a reminder—you are worthy of asking questions. You are not a burden for asking an employee for help!

If in-person shopping is not appealing to you, or your size is not offered in store, the Internet is your happy place. As someone who wears a size that is not always available in store, I am with you! Over the years I have become adept at finding new brands, sizing information, shipping deals, and coupons to allow me to get the most from online shopping. Chances are that you have a lot of this knowledge as well. Now is the time to put it to work! You might even want to start a list to keep track of the stores that have good options for you. There are a bunch of retailers, from big box stores to tiny, online-only brands that carry yoga clothing in inclusive sizing. There are even retailers that will make clothing customized to fit you exactly and give you what you need in terms of technical elements and comfort. Spend some time searching key words that relate to your size, what you're looking for, and the budget you have. You may need to order from a few companies and return what doesn't work for you. This might take a while if your budget is smaller and you need to wait for returns to be processed before you can order from another store. Keep the faith though! Awesome yoga clothes in your size are out there just waiting for you to find them. Here are some brands I've tried and would recommend:

- Superfit Hero (US$$$) makes activewear pieces specifically for plus-size bodies, and the results are high-quality garments that fit well, hold up over time, and are made in the United States. It offers sizes 12-42.
- Rainbeau Curves (US$$) offers activewear and athleisure in fun colors and patterns with sizes from 14-32.
- Universal Standard (US$$$) makes high-quality activewear basics with soft fabrics and strong construction. It offers sizes 00-40.

What to Look For

Not all activewear is created equally! Trust me, I have had my share of split seams, chafing, see-through fabric, immediate pilling, and lots of other annoying and potentially embarrassing problems. The good news is that you can look for certain elements of fabrication that will help you avoid a lot of problems down the road and keep your yoga wardrobe full of clothes that are great looking, fitting, and performing. Spare yourself from wasting money on garments that seem like a good deal or appear well made, but ultimately turn out to be a waste of money. Those yoga pants may be a fun pattern and color, but if they don't last, they're not worth the money!

The first thing to look for with any activewear purchase is a material that both suits your needs and feels nice on your skin. The last thing you want is to have scratchy, itchy, or stiff material distracting you from your yoga practice! Look for material that fits your particular practice's requirements. Are you looking for a natural fiber or something synthetic to wick sweat away? Do you want a technical fabric that's stretchy or a woven material that feels breezy on your skin? Look for materials that feel nice on your skin and you wouldn't mind wearing over and over again. Now is not the time to be uncomfortable! Prioritize getting exactly what you want and need for your practice. Make sure the garment's level of compression matches what you like. I don't particularly enjoy the feeling of high compression, especially around my waist. I look for materials that provide light compression, and even will size up to get a different fit. If you don't have the privilege to size up in a particular brand, look for a different fabrication or try another brand. If you're unhappy and uncomfortable in a garment when trying it on, chances are that you will never wear that item, and it'll be a waste of money.

The second element of a garment I check is the sewing technique on the seams. Most high-quality, tightly fitting activewear is constructed with flatlock seaming. This means that the seams are sewn in a way that helps to prevent them from rubbing on your skin and creating chafing, rashes, or other irritation. This is important for anyone looking for activewear, but especially for folks in bigger bodies! I don't know about you, but preventing chafing is always on my list of must-dos. I have tried yoga pants and tops in the past without flatlock seams that caused major chafing and skin irritation. I consider flatlock seams mandatory for my activewear, but it may be less of a concern for you. You know yourself best and can decide if it's something you want to look out for. In addition to the construction of the seams, you'll want to look for pants designed with a gusset where the two inseams come together. Less expensive pants often do not have this feature, so they will not hold up as well over time. A gusset is a diamond- or square-shaped piece of fabric that's placed where the inseams come together at the crotch of stretchy yoga pants or leggings. It is important because it distributes evenly the strain of stretchy materials pulling to add strength, longevity, and a greater range of movement. Without a gusset, the two inseams would meet each other at the intersection of the front and back seams and create an X that is much less strong and long lasting. I always look to see how a pair of yoga pants is constructed and have found that a pair with a gusset will last much longer and require less maintenance over time.

Regardless of where you find your yoga clothes, remember that you deserve to be comfortable and feel confident. I hope you give yourself permission to wear what feels empowering and to let other people's opinions fall away. If you hesitate to don certain clothing items because you fear judgment from outside, ask yourself what would make you happy. Sometimes choosing to do the thing that scares you is the best way to banish the fear, but sometimes it's not. Take a safe risk if you're feeling bold, but never feel like you have to push yourself to wear, do, or think something that's not authentic to your needs and state of mind. Clothes can be supportive, physically and mentally, but they can also keep you from focusing on your practice if you feel uncomfortable or self-conscious. It all boils down to learning to listen to your body and honoring its needs. It's never a bad decision when you're doing what is right for yourself!

BASIC GEAR FOR A SUPPORTED YOGA PRACTICE

Oh, props, how I've come to love you over the years! Y'all, I can't believe I wasted so much time convincing myself that I didn't need props. Here's what I've learned—everyone needs props. Oh, yes, everyone. From the complete newbie coming into her first pose to a lifelong practitioner who can stand on her head while she sleeps, props make everyone's yoga practice better, more interesting, and more accessible. There's a whole world of yoga-related gear that can enrich your practice and empower you! This section is going to dig into many of the yoga props out there. I want to give you all the information so you can think about what might be helpful and fun to have for your specific practice.

However, let's first take a moment to talk about props in general. What is the point of using them? The short answer is that they help make yoga postures work for your body, but there's a lot more to it. Let's start with the philosophy behind using props. Some folks think of props as a tool that helps you achieve a pose until you're able to do it without that support. This way of thinking reinforces the notion that your body is the problem, which feels very unkind and untrue to me. I bought into this school of thought for a long time and personally suffered because of it. I would not recommend positioning your body as an equation to be solved. Rather, I would hold the pose up as the variable that needs to change. My philosophy about using props is that they are tools to create support, stability, challenge, and interest in postures. Props are not for those who can't. Props are wonderful tools for everyone! Instead of thinking about props as tools you use until you don't have to, try seeing them as helpful resources you get to use to enrich your practice. This shift in perspective takes any judgment out of the equation and allows you to simply celebrate how props can positively affect your practice! You may find that you stop using a certain prop for various poses over time, but you also may not. There's nothing wrong with continuing to use props as you get deeper into your practice. Starting out with this philosophy will serve you well over time and help to contribute to a positive and compassionate relationship with yourself.

Yoga gear can help you build confidence, find support, create accessibility, add layers of challenge, and experience poses in new ways. It gives you the freedom to explore movement, sensation, support, and connection, allowing you to get the full benefit of postures and find new ones along the way. It took me years to realize that my need to prove myself to others by not using props was damaging and counterproductive. All it did was create an adversarial relationship between my mind and body and led me to injure myself, resulting in unnecessary pain and medical expenses. The worst of it all is that it completely counteracted the much-needed mind–body connection benefits that yoga could have brought into my life. Why fight against our bodies and pit them against our minds? Our bodies are neither the enemy nor the problem. It doesn't serve us to punish ourselves by not using the resources available! Meet your body where it is in this moment and give it the support it needs. We have so much to learn from the exploration of options, of difference.

If you're on board with using props, you still might have a lot of questions about which ones are most needed and what kinds are the best. I don't blame you! There are tons of yoga props available these days, and it can be easy to feel overwhelmed. My advice to you is to start with lower-cost basics, and, over time, you can determine if you want to invest in higher-quality and specialized gear. Starting with what you might already have will help to keep costs down if budget is an issue for you. I have lots of suggestions for DIY versions of many of the basic props. It's not necessary to spend a ton of money on expensive gear before you know if you need or want it.

The next section is all about the basic gear I think is most helpful to have as a yoga newbie. I'll talk about each prop's uses, the most common materials you'll find, available sizes, and the price points you might expect. Plus, for each of these, I'll give you tips on DIY versions you can make or household swaps that are good stand-ins. Take care to read through to help you narrow down the list of the props you'd like to gather for your practice.

Yoga Mats

A yoga mat is perhaps the most basic of all the gear you will acquire. These mats serve to create a clean, stable, and safe surface for your practice. It can be a little overwhelming to shop for a mat since they come in many different materials, sizes, and price points. Let's begin with the most common materials you'll find yoga mats are made of: PVC, rubber, and TPE.

PVC, or polyvinyl chloride, is a popular synthetic material, especially in many of the more affordable mats found at big box stores and to rent at studios.

When you think of a standard yoga mat, you're probably picturing a PVC mat. There's a reason they are so widely used, since they tend to be sold at accessible price points. Not all PVC mats are inexpensive though, with high-end brands sometimes choosing to use the material for their products. PVC mats are usually thicker with a long break-in period, but they last a long time and hold up to many years of yoga practices. They provide good traction but can be difficult to keep clean. PVC is not biodegradable, so if that's important to you, look for a mat made of one of the following materials.

Natural rubber mats have gained a lot of popularity, and it's not hard to see why. Rubber is a natural, renewable, and biodegradable material that makes a great yoga mat. If you plan on practicing yoga styles that will leave you very sweaty, a natural rubber mat might be perfect for you! Mats made of rubber provide an extremely stable and safe surface, with lots of grip even at your most sweaty. However, if padding or the thickness of your mat is a high priority, you may want to steer clear of rubber. These mats tend to be a little harder than those made of PVC.

TPE, or thermoplastic elastomer, is a newer synthetic material being used to make yoga mats, and it's becoming pretty popular. Lots of yogis like this material because it's odorless, lightweight, soft, grippy, and biodegradable. The biggest downside to TPE mats is that they don't have the longevity you can get from PVC and natural rubber mats.

Once you decide on a type of material that works best for your needs, you'll need to think about the size. A standard yoga mat is 24 by 68 inches (61 by 173 cm), which can feel small for those of us in larger bodies. It's not necessary, but you can get a mat in a longer length, a wider width, or a combination of both. My first yoga mat was a standard mat I purchased from a big box store, and it felt so small to me! Once I upgraded to an extra-wide, extra-tall mat, I felt more comfortable and supported. I love that mat and still use it today, 15 years later. It's a quarter-inch-thick (0.64 cm) PVC mat, and while it has served me very well at home, I don't choose to bring it with me to classes because it's heavy! Keep in mind that larger mats will weigh more and choose accordingly. While there are lots of sizes of mats available online, not all brands offer these larger sizes. You may have to choose which characteristic is most important to you. I now own three yoga mats that I use at different times. The extra-large PVC one is for home use where weight and size are not limiting factors. I bring a standard-size PVC yoga mat with me to classes if I have to carry it a long way. And I have an extra-long (but not extra-wide) natural rubber mat I take to classes when carrying a heavy mat is not an issue. Obviously you don't need as many yoga mats as I have! Find yourself one good mat to start with and then consider upgrading in the future when you have a good idea of what you want and need from your mat.

There's no reason to go out and purchase a super expensive mat right out of the gate. You may not be sure of which type of mat will work best for your needs, and it seems silly to spend a bunch of money on something that might not be right for you. So, let's talk about prices to give you a better idea of what options are out there. The lower end of the price spectrum will yield standard-size PVC mats for around US$15 to $25. From this point, the prices can range all the way up to US$150 for super-deluxe mats! Often, these high-end mats are more environmentally friendly and durable than less expensive mats. When looking for a mat, especially at the lower end of the price spectrum, don't forget to look at thrift stores, large discount retailers, and online marketplaces. Often you can find good basic yoga mats, still in their packaging, for even less than these prices.

DIY Options

Maybe you want to skip the stores completely and use what you already have. Common household flooring of all sorts can be used safely to practice yoga as long as you're careful and prepared. Hardwood and tile floors can be great for practicing, especially standing poses, as long as you're not wearing slippery socks. If you plan to use your wood or tile floors as your mat, consider investing in a pair of socks with grippy rubber pieces on the bottom as a form of insurance against slipping. Carpet and areas with rugs can work nicely for seated and supine parts of your practice. Standing poses can work also, but take care if your carpet or rug is on the slippery side. If you're going to practice on carpet or a rug, consider going barefoot so you will be less prone to slipping and can feel the ground beneath your feet for stability.

Yoga Blocks

Aside from a mat, the yoga block is probably the most well-known prop there is. Ranging in sizes, materials, and shapes, blocks are helpful tools to bring the floor up to you or find support and stability. Most commonly made from firm foam, wood, or cork, yoga blocks are multitaskers that create a lot of accessibility and support for all levels of yoga practitioners. In this book, you'll find blocks used to create a host of options for supine, seated, and standing poses. They are so versatile and helpful!

Sometimes yoga blocks are used under the hands to bring the floor up to you and make poses more accessible, as seen in the forward-fold or downward-facing dog poses. Other times, the blocks are placed under your body to offer support and relieve strain or help create a stretch, which you see in the bound-angle and supported fish poses. Even more, blocks can be used to help keep you in correct alignment, add a level of challenge, or bring awareness to muscle groups.

The blocks most commonly found in studios and brick-and-mortar retailers are rectangular with dimensions of four by six by nine inches (10 by 15 by 23 cm)—the universal yoga block size that you'll find for sale everywhere. However, it's not the only size of block available to you. Later in the chapter, I'll tell you about some other shapes and sizes of yoga blocks, but, for now, we'll stick to the standard four-inch (10 cm) block. The material of the block is important, especially for using as a support underneath the body. Wood and cork blocks are much harder than their foam counterparts. I personally like foam blocks the best because I find wood and cork versions to be painful to have underneath me in many poses. You might start with foam and see how you tend to use your blocks. It may be that you want the firmer and harder blocks for your particular purposes. Regardless of the material, blocks are incredibly useful and naturally come with three levels: low, medium, and high. The variety of these positions allows blocks to be even more useful because they can adapt to different-sized practitioners, varying poses, and changing needs. Blocks vary in price depending on the material used and brand selling them. Typically, foam blocks are the least expensive, with cork coming in second, and wooden blocks a distant third. Foam blocks can be found for US$5 to $10 at most big box stores, discount retailers, and online yoga stores, and sometimes they pop up at thrift stores. Cork blocks run about US$10 to $20 and are easiest to find at specialty stores and online. Wooden blocks are mostly sold at yoga studios and specialty stores (in-person and online), and you can find them for US$15 to $45.

DIY Options

If you don't want to immediately spend money on yoga blocks, don't worry! There are lots of ways to DIY a stable and strong block alternative at home. If you have some similarly sized books that you don't mind sacrificing, a great hack is to wrap them in paper for protection and then use duct tape all around them to stabilize the stack. If you have the right-sized books, you can make something that performs very much like a block! Also, you can use different-sized stacks to create yoga blocks of varying sizes to perfectly support your practice. Another household swap that's great in a pinch is raiding your pantry for jumbo-sized cans. The standard #10 can is roughly six by seven inches (15 by 18 cm) and provides a very stable base to bring your hands to, though it is not very comfortable for poses requiring you to lean heavily into the can. Stacking unopened reams of printer paper can make a wonderful support for supine poses because the wide, flat nature of the reams is pretty comfortable to position underneath you. For a true DIY, you can use layers of cardboard, cut to size and tightly bound with duct tape, to make your own block in any size or shape. Or hit the hardware store for the free offcuts of wood they leave available for people to grab. A little sandpaper and elbow grease will get you a sturdy wooden block for free! These are a few examples of household swaps or DIY versions of yoga blocks, but there are tons more to be discovered around your house. Get creative and see what you can come up with!

Yoga Blankets

Blankets are an important prop found in most studios and home yogi stashes, and it's not hard to understand why. These thin, tightly woven blankets can be folded and rolled into various shapes to create soft, yet firm, support for a large number of poses. Yoga blankets are a highly versatile prop used not only for support, but also for warmth and a comforting gentle pressure during relaxation practices. These blankets can be folded into a rectangular shape and placed under the hips to make seated positions more comfortable or stacked on each other to create a raised platform to elevate hips, legs, or back. A few good yoga blankets can stand in for a bolster, which we'll talk about in a moment.

When shopping for a yoga blanket, there are a few things to keep in mind. Cotton is a great material that keeps its shape and remains dense enough to support the body when folded or rolled. Be on the lookout for a dense weave without much space in between the threads. Generally, these blankets range from 76 to 84 inches (193 to 213 cm) long by 54 to 66 inches (137 to 168 cm) wide. Many studios sell yoga blankets, but often they're not available at brick-and-mortar big box stores. Some specialty stores will carry blankets, but not all do, so be prepared to head online to find the best choices. Blankets tend to cost around US$10 to $20, but deluxe blankets can be more expensive depending on the materials used and brand name.

DIY Options

Luckily for you, blankets are one of the easiest props to find household swaps for! Many lap-sized blankets sold for use on the couch are well suited for yoga purposes, so you may already have what you need! Beach towels are another excellent stand-in for a yoga blanket, and a large bath towel can work as well. Any tightly woven, semi-thick piece of fabric will take the place of a yoga blanket with ease. Time to raid the linen closet!

Yoga Bolsters

These firm pillows are available in different fabrics and fillings to fit yogis' differing needs. They are incredibly helpful in providing comfort, support, and stretching assistance during restorative postures, long-hold stretches, and deep-breathing exercises. Yoga bolsters come in many different shapes and sizes, but their role is always to give a firm, yet soft, support to help you get the full benefit of your practice. Often, bolsters are placed underneath areas of the body to firmly support your release of tension or to keep you in a certain alignment. Mostly used in restorative yoga, bolsters are helpful any time you're seated or lying on the floor. You don't have to wait for restorative poses to get the benefits of a yoga bolster! Adding the height of a bolster underneath you in many poses can help you experience them in new ways. Often, you can find a new favorite way to experience the pose. Exploring poses is a fun way to keep your practice fresh and new!

Yoga bolsters are most commonly found in cylindrical or rectangular shapes and are offered in many sizes that suit different needs. It's up to you to decide which type is best for your needs, at least in the beginning. You may find yourself hooked on bolsters like me! I currently own four bolsters that I use in different ways depending on my needs. Due to their round shape, cylindrical bolsters are especially good for propping up your knees in deep-relaxation pose. The curved outside fits snugly behind the knees and allows your lower back to release gently toward the floor. Also, cylindrical bolsters are a perfect shape to sit astride for firm, yet yielding, support in hero pose. Rectangular bolsters have a nice, wide flat side to sit on for many seated postures. Depending on the size you choose, the rectangular bolster can lift you off the floor to make sitting cross-legged more comfortable and also give a perfect tilt to your pelvis that makes seated poses more accessible.

You will find a large variety of sizes when shopping for a bolster. Some bolsters are much longer, thicker, or larger all over. For plus-size folks, I recommend purchasing a bolster that is extra firm because, over time, weight can compress standard bolsters to the point of nonfunctionality. I have a deluxe rectangular bolster I use for seated postures that's held its shape extremely well over the years. Other less-firm bolsters I've had didn't hold up well to continued use by me, but your mileage will vary. The thickness of your bolster is another personal preference, with some enjoying the extra height and some preferring a thinner shape. You might experiment at home with the heights of standard bolsters, stacking blankets or firm pillows up to various heights to see which you prefer. Standard rectangular bolsters are approximately 5 to 6 inches (13 to 15 cm) tall, with round bolsters coming in at around 7 to 10 inches (18 to 25 cm) tall. Keep in mind that the bolsters will compress when your body weight is on them. Like the sizes, prices for yoga bolsters vary! Expect to pay US$30 to $50 for a quality bolster. They're not cheap, but bolsters are a wonderful investment if you plan on practicing at home frequently.

DIY Options

If a yoga bolster is out of your budget, consider DIYing your own at home! The first bolster I ever owned was made of random items from around my house, and it has held up for many years! It's not the prettiest bolster in my collection, but it does the job and was entirely free. I didn't follow a pattern; instead, I found small blankets, material scraps, and a wool poncho to roll up and fill a fabric tube I sewed from a bedsheet. I closed the ends . . . and my first bolster was born! If making a yoga bolster isn't in the cards for you, try grabbing firm pillows from your couch, or a stack of thick towels to create a bolster alternative that fits your needs.

Yoga Chairs

Chairs are excellent props for your yoga practice! You can use them to bring support, stability, and accessibility to almost any yoga pose you want to try. While many studios have special metal-folding chairs with the back partially removed, virtually any chair can be a great prop for you. Any material, as long as it's comfortable to touch, will work for a yoga chair. At home, I often use one of my wooden dining room chairs in my practice. What you're looking for in a chair to use for yoga is (1) a sturdy and strong frame, (2) legs without wheels, (3) no arms to get in your way, and (4) your feet can rest firmly on the floor. If your feet don't rest firmly on the floor, don't worry about it! You can use props to find stability and grounding. Dining room chairs are often perfect matches for our requirements.

Using a chair in a yoga practice is often viewed as something for practitioners who are elderly, injured, or have a disability. In fact, yoga chairs are amazing tools for any yoga student! They offer new ways to experience poses and, in some cases, create a more challenging way to practice certain postures. A chair can provide stability in balance poses, accessibility for seated sequences, and support for restorative practices. There are tons of ways to incorporate a chair into your yoga practice that serve to increase the benefits you get and the variety of options available to make your practice fun.

If you'd like to purchase a yoga chair with an open back section, you might be spending US$60 to $100 online. However, if you have a sturdy chair at home, I'd suggest starting with that and seeing how you like it. You can always upgrade later!

DIY Options

The cool thing about yoga chairs is that you probably already have a chair perfectly suited for your practice in your home. Depending on what you're using it for, you might also find your coffee table, couch seat, kitchen counter, or other piece of sturdy furniture to be a great household swap. Take a little tour of your house and look for strong surfaces that might stand in for a chair in a pinch. I love using my kitchen counters as a prop so I can practice yoga while I cook! If you have stairs in your home, you are in luck! There are lots of poses that really benefit from the stability, height adjustments, and support of a few stairs. Be adventurous and see what you have around the house that can help you explore movement and poses!

Yoga Straps

One of the most affordable props is the yoga strap, which is easily found at big box stores, discount retailers, specialty stores, and on many websites for US$5 to $10. These straps come in a few different lengths and materials, and can be very helpful for stretching, support, and accessibility. Yoga straps allow you to extend the length of your arms in order to reach farther, grip more easily, and find the benefit of a pose without straining. Straps can help you maintain control in a pose that otherwise would leave you unstable. Attempting some poses without the help of a yoga strap can put you in incorrect alignment, potentially leading to injury. Straps are easy to use and find and yogis of all experience levels use them to improve the quality of their practice.

Most yoga straps are made of non-stretchy woven cotton, although some are nylon instead. One end will typically have a buckle or other type of closure made of metal or plastic. Straps are often offered in 6, 8, and 10 feet (2 m, 2.5 m, and 3 m), and I personally recommend the longest strap possible. With a 10-foot (3 m) strap, you can do anything you might want to try. Shorter straps are not always long enough for larger bodies to be used in the same ways as straight-sized practitioners. Some yoga straps are stretchy, circular, made of different materials, or consist of loops. There is a whole world of other interesting yoga straps out there, but, in the beginning, a classic strap will serve you best.

DIY Options

Although straps are very affordable, it's also easy to make a DIY version at home or find household swaps to use instead. Any long, sturdy, and flexible piece of non-stretchy material can stand in for a strap! Woven belts, robe ties, or neckties joined together can work in a pinch. A thin, rolled-up beach towel is also a good alternative, as is a nylon-woven dog leash that's long enough. Chances are good that you have a great strap alternative in your home already!

YOGA PROPS DEEP DIVE

While sticking with the basics is encouraged, there are tons of really interesting specialized gear that can also add to your yoga practice. The items listed in this section are not even everything that's out there, but they are some of my personal favorite items. It may be a long time before you find yourself interested in adding new props to your setup, but go ahead and peruse the list anyway. You might find something you'd like to try!

Blocks of Other Sizes and Shapes

While the standard four-inch (10 cm) rectangular block is an amazing tool, there are a variety of other types available to you. You can find wide, flat rectangular shapes that are great for stacking to create the perfect height, wedge-shaped blocks to relieve wrist strain and help with inversions, giant 13-inch-tall (33 cm) super blocks for incredibly stabilizing and accessible support, rounded-edged blocks for ergonomics, and even egg-shaped blocks made to fit the body's curves.

Eye Pillows

Eye pillows are small fabric pillows filled with flax seeds, rice, or other small, lightweight materials. When placed over the eyes in relaxation postures, the pillows provide total light blocking and a gentle weighted feeling on the eyes. This gentle pressure on the eyes stimulates the vagus nerve, which can help lower heart rate and regulate your mood.

Rubber Massage Balls

I have an intense love for rubber massage balls! They've been key players in helping me recover from injuries, muscle tension and soreness, and all kinds of pain. While you can purchase yoga massage balls, you can save some money by getting three- to four-inch (8 to 10 cm) solid rubber bouncy balls online. For about a quarter of the price of balls made for yoga or acupressure massage, you can get an effective ball that works exactly the same way as a specific yoga ball. A great time to break out the balls and massage yourself is after your yoga practice when your body is warm and ready to stretch.

Meditation Cushions or Pranayama Bolsters

Meditation cushions and pranayama bolsters are not the same thing, but I've grouped them together because they're both other types of firm pillows that can be helpful to yoga practitioners. Meditation cushions are thick, round pillows stuffed with firm batting that make sitting on the floor for longer periods of time more comfortable. While they're great for meditation, they can be used for your yoga asana practice as well. They are as useful for support and cushioning as standard yoga bolsters.

Pranayama bolsters are also helpful tools for making yourself more comfortable on the floor. Named after one of the eight limbs of yoga, pranayama bolsters are smaller than standard yoga bolsters and create a comfy seat for practicing breath work.

Kneepads

A folded blanket will serve you well to provide cushioning and protection for your knees and sacrum. If you typically have problems with kneeling or lying on the floor, you may consider adding a special kneepad to your gear list. There are some yoga-specific kneepads out there, but gardening pads work just as well and tend to be less expensive.

Yoga Towels

If you plan on practicing highly energetic forms of yoga that leave you dripping in sweat, a yoga towel would be handy to own. Yoga towels come in different sizes and usually are made of microfiber fabric that soaks up sweat without becoming slippery. Many practitioners of power yoga, hot yoga, and vinyasa yoga swear by the mat-sized towels they lay down and perform their entire practice on. These large towels keep them from slipping around on their mats.

Yoga Wheels

These props are sometimes intimidating for folks new to them, but they are very simple to use. Yoga wheels are strong, circular props usually covered in a layer of foam similar to a PVC yoga mat. You can use these to help stretch and support your back, to stand on to add extra challenge to your balance poses, or to experience poses in new ways.

Headstand Helpers

While headstand helpers come in many forms, they are commonly used as some type of support for your shoulders that help you come into and remain in headstand pose. Often, headstand helpers are made of a wooden base with padding where your shoulders sit. If you plan on working toward a headstand, a headstand helper can be very useful as you gain confidence and strength.

Sandbags

A sandbag is exactly what it sounds like! Sandbags are used in restorative yoga poses to add weight to various body parts to create more stretch, grounding, or sensation in those areas. Generally weighing between 7 and 10 pounds, sandbags are often used at studios and sometimes at home. I have a sandbag and love placing it on my pelvis in relaxation poses or on my shoulders in seated forward-folds to help me move closer to the floor.

CONCLUSION

Perhaps now that you've arrived at the end of this chapter, you're feeling knowledgeable and ready to start pulling your gear together. Or maybe, instead, you're feeling overwhelmed and still confused about what you need to get started. Don't worry, you're doing just great no matter how you're feeling right now! In fact, this is a perfect time to practice mindfulness! If you're not familiar, mindfulness asks us to pay attention without passing judgment. This can mean to notice other people and situations without moving on to judge them, and it also refers to not judging yourself for your feelings and sensations. Feeling excited and feeling overwhelmed are both temporary states of being, and neither of them deserves your judgment. Take a moment to connect with your emotions and practice noticing without judgment. Then you can rationally move onto the next right step for you. This may be moving forward with purchasing or DIYing props for your yoga practice. However, it might mean taking more time to research and think about what are the best gear purchases for you. Give yourself permission to not have an answer in this moment! There's plenty of time to figure it out as we move along.

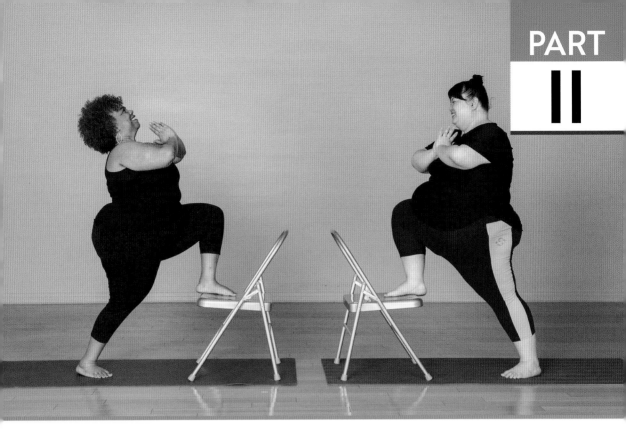

Get Moving

CHAPTER 3

WARMING UP AND BREATHING EXERCISES

Like any type of movement you might try out, yoga requires a warm-up to keep you safe and prepare the body for the postures to come. Depending on your focus for that day, a warm-up might focus specifically on certain areas of the body or on prepping all parts. It's helpful to think about what your body needs and wants when you start to warm up. If time isn't limited, try to warm up your whole body to give every part some attention and help increase the blood flow to all your muscles. If you're running short on time, just focus on warming up the parts of your body directly affected by the postures you're going to practice. However, keep in mind that your body is a network of connected muscles, tendons, and ligaments. Without a proper warm-up, it's easy to increase the likelihood of being sore the next day and even injure yourself. It's safest to practice a warm-up that gets your whole body ready to hit the mat and enjoy some movement.

In this chapter, we'll explore some great ways to warm up your body, from fingers and toes to your spine and hips. Many small movements and stretches can prepare your body for whatever comes next. I'll talk about options you can do from a seated position on the floor or in a chair, as well as some done while standing. No matter what kind of yoga practice you have planned, there is a simple warm-up that can get your body ready in just a few minutes.

I'll also discuss how to sit comfortably on the floor without falling over or cutting circulation off in your legs. There are tons of adjustments, supportive props, and alternative postures that can make dealing with seated poses and stretches much more comfortable and accessible. We'll look at some of those and also talk about ways to support yourself in getting up and down from the floor whether you're at home or in a class with others. Sometimes it's easy to talk ourselves into just dealing with the pain, inconvenience, and potential injury that comes with ignoring our body's needs. I know from personal experience how tempting it can be to act like you don't need support, assistance, or different options than other students. I hope you're learning to trust that I won't steer you wrong! Let me help you find options and support to make your yoga practice happier and healthier for you in the long run.

SITTING COMFORTABLY ON THE FLOOR

Oh, man, you wouldn't believe how many times I've heard people talk about the difficulty they have in sitting comfortably on the floor! It's got to be one of the most discussed topics for folks new to yoga, and with good reason. Sitting on the floor is incredibly uncomfortable for many people, not just folks in bigger bodies, though you wouldn't know it from looking at yoga in magazines or on TV. All we're shown are super flexible people gliding smoothly onto the floor into pretzel-like positions with ease. What they don't show us is the struggle many people have staying upright in a seated position and how to not lose circulation in your legs while you're there.

There are lots of reasons why sitting on the floor might suck for you, but some of the most commonly experienced are (1) your belly hits your thighs and keeps you from being able to sit upright easily, so you strain to stay up, (2) your hamstrings are tight, which turns staying upright into an ab workout, and (3) a variety of muscles in the hips and inner thighs are tight and make it difficult to be upright on the floor. Don't worry though! There are easy ways to make sitting on the floor more comfortable and accessible, and we'll get into them right now.

Raise Your Hips

My first question to those who have trouble sitting on the floor is to ask whether or not they've tried sitting up on a bolster, block, or folded blanket(s). Sitting up on some kind of support raises the hips and changes the angles of your body. In general, the higher you raise your hips, the easier it feels to sit on the floor. Try it right now! Grab a small blanket or super firm pillow and sit down on it, your hips scooted close to the front edge. You want your butt on the support, not your thighs. How does it feel?

Depending on your body, you might choose to use a softer or firmer support underneath you. You might choose a low, folded blanket or a higher support that combines items for a taller seat. Experiment and see what feels best for your body. There's no one way to do this, so let yourself try different versions. You may find that one style of raising your hips works best for a cross-legged seat, and another is better for a wide-leg position. Prioritize your comfort! Don't be afraid to change what you're doing if it's no longer working for you.

Switch Your Leg Position

The next question I ask folks with floor-sitting woes is what position they've been using. Often, we're instructed to sit with the soles of the feet together or legs crossed, and that's just not comfortable for lots of people. It may sound basic, but changing your leg position might be the key to being comfy on the floor! A combination of sitting up on a support to raise the hips and changing your leg position can completely change how it feels to sit on the floor.

Let's explore some leg positions commonly used to sit on the floor comfortably. I want to start with my absolute favorite way to sit on the floor: soles of the feet together with hips open and knees out to each side. This position, the foundation for bound-angle pose, is my go-to sitting position because it makes room for my belly and feels very grounding. Others find it more comfortable to sit cross-legged, especially when raising the hips as well. Other great options are to bring the legs wide out to each side for a wide-leg position. This is a great way to feel stable and grounded since there's so much contact with the floor under each leg and your hips. If straight knees are uncomfortable here, place a block or folded blanket under each knee or thigh to give support to the knee joints. Also part of the wide-leg family is a great position I love to sit in on the floor: Keep one leg out wide and bring the other in toward the center, pulling the foot in toward your groin. This position is a great way to work on hip flexibility, one side at a time. Be sure to switch legs so that both hips get a chance to stretch.

There are plenty more leg positions that are options for you to try out when you're on the floor, but these are some of my personal favorites that have also been helpful for my students. The best way to figure out what works for you is to experiment! Give it a go; try out some different leg positions and see how they feel. Don't forget to raise your hips with support and always listen to your body. You'll know very quickly if a position isn't right for you. Bodies are great at telling us to knock it off! We just have to listen to them!

Move Your Belly

People are often uncomfortable talking about or touching their bellies, even when alone. I understand how that feels because I spent a lot of my life feeling the same way. This section might make you uncomfortable, but hear me out and give it a shot. Adjusting your belly might be a revelation for you the way it was for me! It never occurred to me that I could reach down and move my belly to make sitting on the floor or practicing poses more accessible. It sounds SO SIMPLE, but I was never encouraged to connect with my belly in any way except for wishing it were gone. My training with Abby Lentz of HeavyWeight Yoga and Anna Guest-Jelley of Curvy Yoga taught me that touching my belly, adjusting it, and moving it was a wonderful way to make poses work for me in ways I literally had not imagined! I hope that this section might bring you a little of that magic. You can touch your belly! You can pick it up and move it into a better position to make sitting more comfortable, get deeper into a stretch, or bring your body into better alignment.

Touching your belly is not only helpful in moving it into a better position but also affirming; it's a nice way to add reassuring connection into your practice. Here are a couple of ways to touch your belly and adjust its position for comfort, depth, and alignment. You'll probably need to experiment with these two options to find what works best for you in each new situation. Or maybe you'll find a different way to adjust your belly that's even better!

The first technique I want to explain is the one I most often turn to for creating space, sitting more comfortably, and deepening a stretch. It involves bringing your right hand to the right side of your lower belly and gently cupping the curve with your fingers underneath. Then slide your hand and belly to the left until your belly sits closer to the center of your body. Your right thigh should hold this side of your belly in place until you change leg positions. Bring the left hand to the left side of your lower belly and repeat the actions to the opposite side. Your belly should now sit toward the center with extra space available for easier upright sitting and forward folding.

The second technique is great for making space available underneath your belly because the thighs can come together. This is especially helpful when seated with legs straight out to the front. Begin by reaching both hands underneath your belly and lifting it straight up away from your thighs. Arrange your legs in whatever position you want, and then gently place your belly on top of your thighs. It can rest here until you're ready to change leg positions.

These two are just a couple of examples of how adjusting your belly can create space and a more comfortable position. My advice here is the same as before—experiment! Try out a combination of support under your hips, different leg positions, and moving your belly. I know you'll find some great ways to make the floor suck less!

Skip the Floor Altogether!

While I encourage you to continue to work on flexibility and finding the right options to make sitting on the floor comfortable, there's another strategy we haven't discussed yet: Just don't sit on the floor. There are ways to make any pose or stretch accessible to you from a chair, and there is no reason to not allow yourself to take this option. You may have a knee-jerk reaction to this suggestion and immediately want to pass, but hear me out. Often, the reason accessible options aren't taken seriously is because our culture has taught us that they are lesser options to be taken only when you can't do it any other way. As we discussed in the chapter about props, that's silly! Accessibility is not just for those who can't. Accessible options are interesting and valid options that can enrich anyone's practice. Trying new approaches is how we learn and grow. It helps us to be compassionate and knowledgeable about what it's like to take these options. And it's a great way to mix it up and keep your practice fresh.

Consider trying out seated postures and stretches from a chair to see what it feels like. You can experiment with finding support while sitting in a chair by placing a bolster or blocks under your feet or behind your back (see figure

3.1*a*). You can even use multiple chairs to come into a wide-leg position by placing each foot onto a chair and sliding them apart (see figure 3.1*b*). You may find a new favorite way to move and stretch! Other options that don't involve being seated on your butt on the floor are kneeling or sitting on a low stool or meditation bench or cushion.

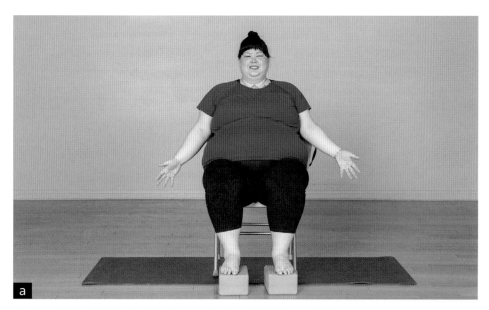

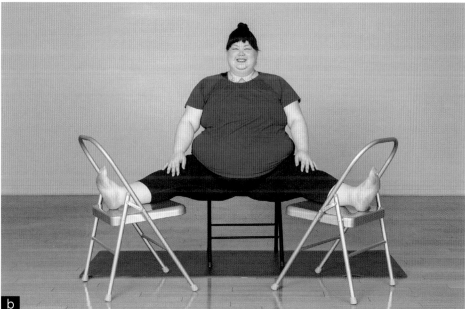

Figure 3.1 Chair options: *(a)* with support under the feet; *(b)* with three chairs to support a wide-leg position.

GETTING UP AND DOWN FROM THE FLOOR

Another challenge many folks face is getting up and down from the floor. It's not surprising that this is a problem since we don't tend to practice this very often in regular life. Then all of a sudden it's time for yoga and our teachers want us to get up and down a hundred times during class. No thank you! Not that I think we shouldn't work on functional flexibility and mobility, but too often, rapidly moving between standing and sitting doesn't take into account people's needs for support and accessibility. Even the most able-bodied folks can benefit from using support and being mindful in their movements. The following are a few sources of support that can make getting up and down from the floor easier and safer.

Blocks

The simple boost of using blocks can make the process of transitioning between up and down much easier. Blocks bring the floor up to you and can make it easier to feel supported as you come down to the floor and back up again. Try turning the blocks to different heights to find the perfect support for you. Hold the blocks in your hand and, with bent knees, fold forward and reach the blocks to the floor. Settle the blocks firmly and bring one knee down and then the other. Find a comfortable seated position. When you're ready to come up, bring your hands to the blocks and work yourself to your knees. Tuck the toes and lift one and then the other knee and gently work yourself up to standing, keeping your knees bent.

Wall

A wall is a great prop to use, especially when blocks and other props are not available. You can count on the sturdiness of a wall to be supportive as you come up and down from the floor. Start with your hands on the wall and bend your knees as you come down to the floor. Keeping contact with the wall, walk your hands down as you kneel and find a comfortable seated position. Don't be afraid to really lean into the wall! It can take your weight and is a great support.

Chair

A chair is very helpful when it comes to finding support for moving up and down from the floor. You can begin with hands on the back of the chair and slowly move down until your hands are on the chair seat. As you bend your knees and come down to the floor, you can move your hands to wherever they need to be to get the best support. Coming up from the floor is similar, with the chair seat being the first stop for your hands and then the chair back as you move higher. Also, don't forget that a very real and valid option is to choose not to come to the floor at all! Feel free to take a seat in a chair for the seated poses and stretches. Honoring your body's needs is powerful self-care!

GENTLE STRETCHES AND MOVEMENTS TO LOOSEN AND WARM THE BODY

Warming up the body in preparation for your practice is so important for your safety! Launching straight into more intense stretches, twists, and other poses is a recipe for injury that's easily avoided with some simple gentle stretches and movements. Start with wrists, hands, and fingers; move to feet and ankles; and then neck and shoulders. Once you've gotten the ball rolling with those, it's time for a little more movement and warming of the spine, hips, and legs. There are many fun warm-up sequences you can put together, but this is a great jumping-off point. If you practice these, you'll be ready for more movement and stretching, and you'll know your body is properly prepared.

Wrists and Hands

Your wrists, hands, and fingers work constantly to help you type, text, and function in so many ways, but are often ignored.

Instruction

▥ Start by rotating your wrists in figure-eight motions, finding your range of motion and checking in with how your forearms, wrists, and hands are feeling.

▥ Then, move back and forth between squeezing your hands into tight fists and releasing them, and follow it up by gently shaking your hands and fingers.

▥ Finally, bring one palm up and one down and place the downward-facing thumb over the other and gently press down. Repeat the gentle press with each finger of the downward-facing hand, being sure to hold long enough to get a good stretch (see figure 3.2). When you've finished one hand, switch and begin again with the other hand in the downward-facing position. By the end, you should have pressed each downward-facing finger gently into its counterpart on the upward-facing hand and given them all a nice stretch.

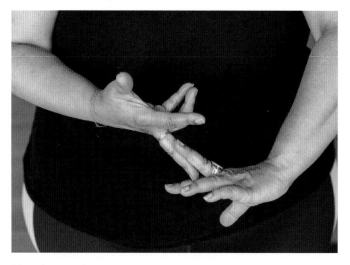

Figure 3.2 Hand stretch.

Ankles and Feet

Oh, wow, is there a section of your body that works as hard and gets less love and attention? I think not! Our ankles and feet work overtime to help us get around, balance, and move. What do we do to thank them? Shove them into uncomfortable shoes and complain about them when they start to hurt. This part of the warm-up is a great time to send a little gratitude and appreciation to your ankles and feet.

Instruction

- Sit on a chair or on the floor with your legs out straight and long. Flex your feet (see figure 3.3*a*), bending at the ankles and pulling your toes back to intensify the stretch. You should feel a stretch up the backs of your legs and maybe even some activity in the fronts of your ankles.
- Point your toes (see figure 3.3*b*), pressing them away from you and stretching across the tops of your feet. Move back and forth between flexing and pointing your feet a few times.
- Roll your ankles in circles in both directions, a few times each way.
- Now it's time for the hitchhiker (see figure 3.3*c*), a toe movement that stretches your toes and feet. With your feet relaxed, flex your big toes and point the other four away. This will probably feel weird the first few times you practice it, but, in time, you could see relief of foot pain, better balance, and fewer foot cramps in standing poses.
- Switch to the other guy (see figure 3.3*d*), the opposite toe movement where the big toes point away and the other four flex up. If you start to feel a foot cramp coming on, just wiggle your toes a lot, and it should stop. Move back and forth between the two toe movements a couple of times before wiggling your toes and rolling your ankles again.

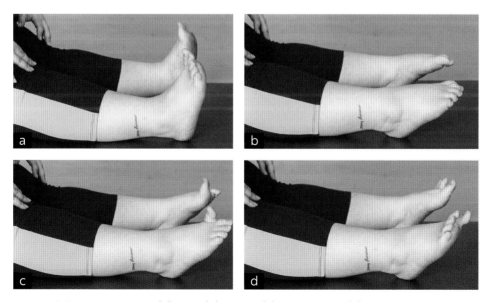

Figure 3.3 Foot series: *(a)* flex; *(b)* point; *(c)* hitchhiker; *(d)* other guy.

Neck and Shoulders

Our necks and shoulders take the brunt of a lot of our anxiety and tension, which can lead to uncomfortably tight muscles and back pain. A great way to work on these pains is to include neck and shoulder stretches in your gentle warm-up. There are many more options available to you for neck and shoulder stretching, but this series is a great place to start. I practice this almost every day, and it really helps me keep my shoulders and neck feeling great!

Instruction: Neck

- Bring your left ear to your left shoulder and let the right arm rest gently on the floor by your side or just hang if you're in a chair. Let gravity press your right shoulder and head down in opposite directions (see figure 3.4a).
- Keeping the sideways tilt of your head, bring your chin up toward the ceiling for a few breaths (see figure 3.4b). Then, keeping the tilt of your head, bring your chin down toward the floor for a few breaths (see figure 3.4c). Finally, return the ear to your shoulder for a few more breaths.
- Bring your head to the center and look left and right, finding your range of motion for today. Then, bring the right ear to the right shoulder and repeat the previous steps on this side.
- Bring your head to the center and drop the chin to your chest, stretching the back of the neck long. Raise your chin up to the ceiling, keeping space between the back of your head and your neck so that your neck stays long. Stretch your chin up and away, moving from the center to the left and right sides. You may even choose to slide your jaw forward to give yourself an underbite and stretch the front of your neck (see figure 3.4d).
- Bring your head back to the center and make any gentle movements of your head and neck that feel good.

Instruction: Arm Rotations

- Bring your arms out to each side (see figure 3.5a).
- Rotate from the shoulders to bring your arms around and up so that the palms face up.
- Bring the arms forward and reverse your twisting to bring your palms to face down or even out (see figure 3.5b). Think of wringing a mop out as you twist from the shoulders to the fingertips.
- Continue rotating back and forth to find your shoulders' range of motion today.

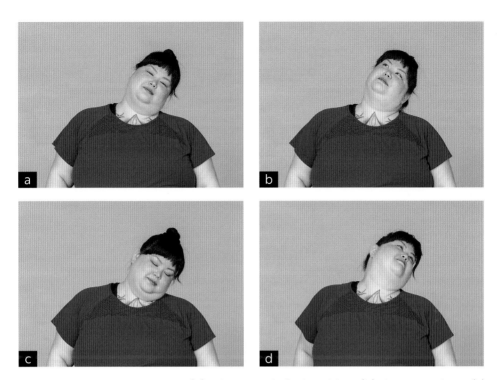

Figure 3.4 Neck stretches: *(a)* left ear to left shoulder; *(b)* chin to ceiling; *(c)* chin to floor; *(d)* chin up to ceiling and over to the side.

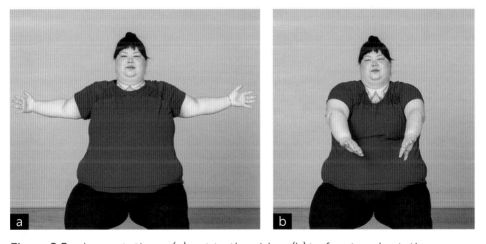

Figure 3.5 Arm rotations: *(a)* out to the sides; *(b)* to front and rotating.

Instruction: Shoulder Stretches

▓ Hold the arms overhead or up in a high V with the palms facing forward. Press your hands back until you feel a stretch in the front of your shoulders and across your chest (see figure 3.6a).

▓ With your hands remaining back, slide your arms down until they're straight out to the sides (see figure 3.6b) and then down into a low V (see figure 3.6c). Hold here and try lifting the chest up toward the ceiling for a small backbend.

▓ Bring your chest back to center and, keeping the hands pressed back, slide your arms back to the sides and finally up to the starting position.

▓ Move the arms to the front of your body, straight out from your chest, with palms together. Straighten your arms and slide your hands forward until you feel a stretch across your shoulder blades and upper back (see figure 3.6d).

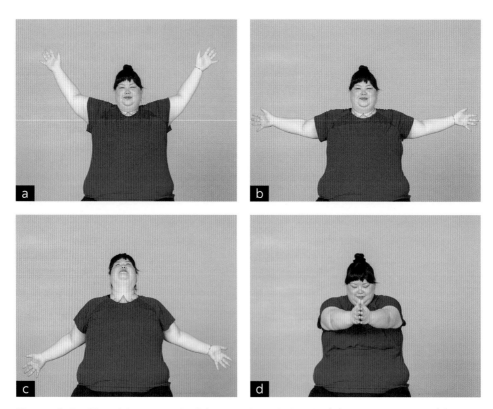

Figure 3.6 Shoulder stretch: (a) press hands back; (b) arms to sides; (c) arms in low V; (d) arms forward, palms together.

Forward-Fold

There are lots of ways to prepare your body for more movement and stretching. I encourage you to try several of them and find what works best for you. One of my favorites is to do a series of forward-folds in a seated or standing position. Forward-folds, especially when moving in time with your breath, are a perfect way to warm up your spine, hips, and legs. They can get your muscles and joints ready for more and also start to get blood moving and breath flowing. Forward-folds are really adaptable, and you can do them seated on the floor, seated on a chair, and standing. I'll talk about each of these ways, and you can try them out to see how each one feels in your body.

Instruction: Seated on the Floor

- Find a comfortable seated position on the floor where you don't strain to stay upright. I find bringing soles of the feet together with hips open and knees out to the side to be nice for forward folding. Also, a great leg position for many folks is to have the legs out wide in a V. However, don't feel that you need to limit yourself to just these leg positions! Try these forward-folds in various leg positions to see what works best for your body and remember that our needs are always changing. Mix things up to keep your practice fresh and give your body what it needs.

- From your seated position, inhale and raise arms overhead while lifting your torso up long from the waist (see figure 3.7*a*).

- Exhale and hinge forward from the hips to bring arms out to the front and down toward the ground (see figure 3.7*b*). Keep your spine straight and your shoulders back, leading with your chest.

- When you reach the point on your way down where you can't keep your back straight any longer, allow the shoulders to come forward (see figure 3.7*c*). Continue the fold, rounding your spine, and let your arms rest down onto the floor or your legs.

- You can either hold here for a few breaths or continue to move with your breath and roll up gently on your next inhale. Repeat as many times as you like, or until your body feels ready to move on.

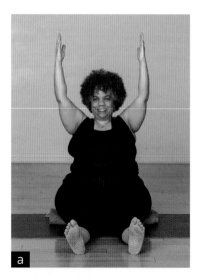

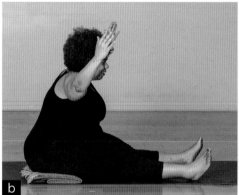
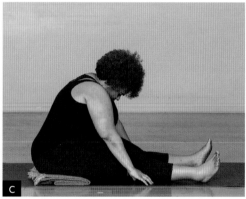

Figure 3.7 Seated forward-fold: *(a)* reach up; *(b)* lean forward with a flat back; *(c)* round over.

Instruction: Seated on a Chair

■ Find a sturdy chair that has no wheels or arms and place it on a nonslip surface or up against a wall. It's important to always check the position of your chair when using it for yoga. It's easy to injure yourself if your chair slides on the floor or isn't sturdy to begin with.

■ Slide forward in your chair until your thighs are mostly off the seat. If you need back support, you can place a pillow or block behind you. Proper posture in your chair is really important for alignment and safety reasons. Make sure your feet can firmly press into the floor to ground you and give you support in your forward-folds. If your feet don't easily reach the floor, try putting blocks or a firm bolster under them.

■ Your legs can be straight out to the front and close together or wider apart to make space for your belly. I prefer a wider leg position when practicing forward-folds from a chair. Try it both ways and see what you think!

▥ From your seated position, inhale and raise your arms overhead while lifting your torso up long from the waist (see figure 3.8*a*).

▥ Exhale and hinge forward from the hips to bring arms out to the front and down toward the ground. Keep your spine straight and your shoulders back, leading with your chest (see figure 3.8*b*). Pay attention to your hips; keep them firmly grounded to the chair seat. It's easy to forget about them and find yourself tipping forward and coming out of alignment or even falling out of your chair. Ask me how I know!

▥ When you reach the point on your way down where you can't keep your back straight any longer, allow the shoulders to come forward. Continue the fold, rounding your spine, and let your arms rest down onto the floor or your legs (see figure 3.8*c*).

▥ You can either hold here for a few breaths or continue to move with your breath and roll up gently on your next inhale. Repeat as many times as you like, or until your body feels ready to move on.

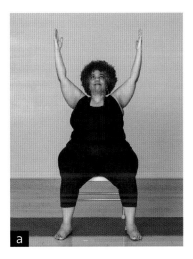

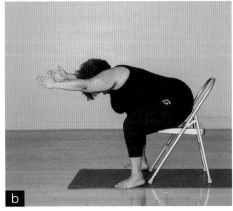 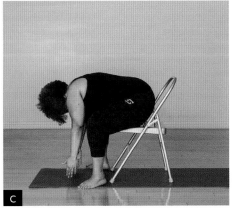

Figure 3.8   Chair forward-fold: *(a)* lift arms overhead; *(b)* hinge forward, leading with the chest; *(c)* round the spine.

Instruction: Standing

▦ To practice forward-folds from standing, bring your feet a comfortable distance apart. This can mean feet are close together or wider apart; both feet positions are great for forward-folds! For the warm-up, I like to perform forward-folds with my legs wider. Then, once I'm feeling a little more loose and warmed up, I will bring my feet closer together for a few more forward-folds. This way, I gently ease the backs of my legs into the stretching, and it feels nicer. That's just my opinion, though, and I encourage you to experience this for yourself and find your favorite ways to practice standing forward-folds.

▦ From your grounded standing position, inhale and raise arms up overhead while lifting your torso up long from the waist. Press down through your legs and feet into the floor to ground yourself (see figure 3.9*a*).

▦ Keeping a slight bend, or softness, in your knees, exhale and hinge forward from the hips. Bring your arms out to the front and down toward the ground. Keep your spine straight and your shoulders back, leading with your chest (see figure 3.9*b*).

▦ When you reach the point on your way down where you can't keep your back straight any longer, allow the shoulders to come forward and round. Continue the fold, rounding your spine, and let your arms rest down onto the floor or a block (see figure 3.9*c*).

▦ Once you're down, play with straightening your knees any amount to feel the stretch up the back of your legs. Be gentle with yourself! Don't force your knees to straighten all the way if they don't want to. Just straighten them enough to stretch the backs of your legs.

▦ You can either hold here for a few breaths or continue to move with your breath and roll up gently on your next inhale. Be sure to keep your knees soft or slightly bent as you come up. Repeat as many times as you like, or until your body feels ready to move on.

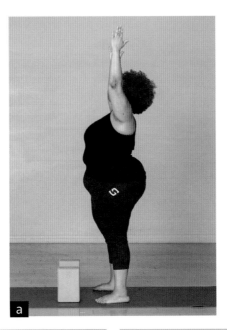

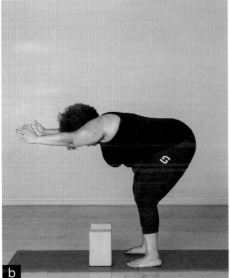

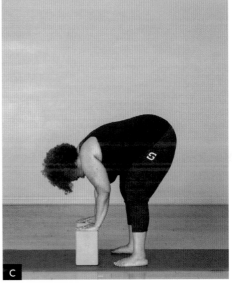

Figure 3.9 Standing forward-fold: *(a)* lift arms overhead; *(b)* hinge at hips and fold forward; *(c)* round shoulders and spine.

BASIC BREATHING TECHNIQUES

The yogic practice of breathing with intention, or pranayama, is as important to your yoga practice as physical postures or meditation. In fact, these breathing techniques can act as a bridge between physical and mental parts of your yoga practice. Pranayama is often used to bring yourself into a meditative state, to become present in your body, and to regulate your mood or energy. If all of this sounds a little woo-woo for you, don't worry. There's actual science behind these claims! A quick search online can bring up studies and anecdotal evidence showing that breath work can help improve lung capacity; reduce blood pressure; and reduce the symptoms of stress, anxiety, depression, and insomnia.

I haven't always had the strongest breath work practice, and it's easy to overlook how important it is. When I started experimenting with different types of breathing techniques, I found myself more able to regulate my mood, with increased lung capacity, and having more fun in my yoga practice. I'd like to remind you of something that's always helpful for me to hear. Yoga is more than just the physical postures, though that's what we see most of online and in the media. You could have a strong yoga practice for the rest of your life and hardly ever do any postures. There are seven other limbs on the tree of yoga, and pranayama is one of them. If you find your mind getting stuck on the physical form of yoga, take some breaths and remember that there is so much more for you to explore. We are not tied to asana, the postures, for an impactful practice. Breath work can be transformative! I'd like to share some of my favorite breathing techniques with you. These are the ones that I call on when I'm in need of grounding, centering, calming, energizing, or to help me get through a challenging time.

Calming, Grounding, and Meditative Breathing

These breathing techniques are my go-to pranayama practices when I'm feeling the need to connect with the earth, my body, and my breath. They bring in extra oxygen, switch my focus to the internal, and create opportunities for me to become grounded in my surroundings and myself. Be gentle with yourself when trying a new breathing technique. It's easy to get frustrated if you feel like you're not getting the hang of it. Keep trying and be kind to yourself! You'll get it eventually and will be able to practice and use the benefits forever.

Alternate Nostril Breathing (Nadi Shodhana)

This is my absolute favorite and most practiced type of pranayama! It is so good at facilitating relaxation, calm, and ease in my body and mind.

Instruction

- To practice, come to a comfortable seated position where you are supported and can bring all your focus to your breath. While other breathing techniques can be practiced lying down, I wouldn't recommend it for this particular type of breath work. This technique requires holding your arm in a raised position for the length of the practice. If you have difficulty holding it up for that long or just would like some support, place a bolster across your legs and use it to support your elbow.

- Begin by closing your right nostril by gently pressing it with your thumb (see figure 3.10a). Inhale through your left nostril, and then close it with your ring finger or little finger (see figure 3.10b).

- Release your thumb to open the right nostril and slowly exhale (see figure 3.10c).

- Keeping the right nostril open, inhale, then gently close it again with your thumb.

- Open your left nostril and slowly exhale. This is considered one cycle of the breath. You can repeat as many times as you like, but perhaps, in the beginning, try it for three to five cycles of the breath.

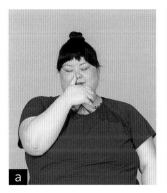 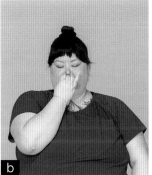 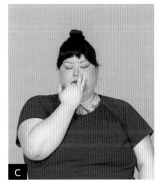

Figure 3.10 Alternate nostril breathing: *(a)* close right nostril with thumb; *(b)* inhale through left nostril, then close it with finger; *(c)* release thumb to open right nostril and exhale.

Three-Part Breathing (Dirga Pranayama)

This breathing technique is an excellent introduction to yogic breath work. The three-part breath is commonly used at the beginning of class as a warm-up and at the end of class as a way to bring yourself back into connection with your body and breath. It's a great way to practice how to fully fill and empty your lungs and can be helpful for those who have trouble staying present in their bodies during pranayama. During the three-part breath, you'll take big breaths of air, which will help to expand your lung capacity. This type of breathing is really helpful for me in relieving stress and anxiety. I hope it will be for you also!

Instruction

- To get started, sit in a comfortable position or lie on your back on the floor or in bed. Let your face and body relax so that your focus is on your breath.
- Begin by inhaling and exhaling deeply through the nose, filling your lungs and expanding your belly like a balloon.
- With each exhale, send all the air from your lungs up and out through your nose. As your belly contracts on your exhale, pull your belly button back toward your spine as if you were pressing and pushing all the air out of a balloon.
- Repeat this deep-belly breathing for a few breaths until you're comfortable with the expanding and contracting technique in the belly. This is the first phase of the three-part breath.
- On your next inhale, expand your belly like before. Then, continue the inhale and create a similar expansion in your rib cage, causing the muscles between your ribs to stretch.
- With each exhale, send all the air from your lungs up and out through your nose. Relax your rib cage so that the ribs slide closer together and then relax your belly, pulling your belly button back toward your spine.
- Repeat these deep inhales and exhales that begin at the ribs and continue to the belly until you feel comfortable with this second phase of the three-part breath.
- When you're ready to move on, inhale deeply, expanding first the belly, then the ribs, and adding in the chest.
- With each exhale, send all the air from your lungs up and out through your nose. First, release the breath from your chest, then relax your rib cage so the ribs slide closer together, and then finally, your belly can release as you pull your belly button back toward your spine.
- Practice this third phase, with all parts of the breath coming together smoothly. Inhale and expand from the belly, moving up to the ribs and then the chest. Exhale and release the breath and any tension from the chest down to the ribs and then the belly.

Box Breath (Sama Vritti)

This breathing technique, sometimes called square breathing, can be a powerful relaxation tool to clear your mind, relax your body, and allow you to focus on being present in your body. It's a favorite of mine to teach in class because it's easy to explain and very effective. It's built on the idea of giving equal attention to all four parts of your breath. This includes (1) the inhale, (2) the pause between inhale and exhale, (3) the exhale, and (4) the pause between exhale and inhale. Normally, we focus on the inhale and the exhale only, but this breath asks you to honor all parts equally. You can practice this seated on the floor, in a chair, or lying down. The details of how to practice this are pretty flexible. You can choose a length of breath that works for you, as long as you feel comfortable and not panicked or short of breath. For the explanation here, I've chosen a length of four counts, but you can tailor this to your own needs every time you practice.

Instruction

- Inhale slowly through your nose for four counts. Notice what it feels like to inhale and fill your lungs.
- At the top of your inhale, full of air, hold for four counts before beginning your exhale. Try to think of it as just not exhaling rather than specifically holding your breath. As you hold, you can investigate what it feels like to hold, full of air.
- Exhale slowly through your nose for four counts.
- At the bottom of your exhale, emptied of air, hold for four counts before beginning your inhale. Try to think of it as just not inhaling rather than specifically holding your breath. As you hold, you can investigate what it feels like to hold, emptied of air.
- Continue breathing, giving equal time and attention to all four parts of your breath for five minutes or until you feel calm and grounded.

Energizing Breathing

The following breathing techniques are my most used pranayama practices for when I need to increase my energy, perk up my mood, or get myself moving. These practices help to oxygenate my blood, warm my body, and inspire me to move my body more. Try to practice these for a few minutes at a time and check in with yourself to see how you feel. If it feels uncomfortable to breathe in these ways, allow yourself to feel that discomfort. Give yourself permission to try them a few times and get the hang of the techniques. These are favorites of mine, but that doesn't mean they'll be favorites of yours!

Ocean Breath (Ujjayi)

This is one of the first breathing techniques I learned, and it remains one of my most used breath practices. Ujjayi breath can both energize and relax me, and this versatility is one of the reasons I love it. This way of breathing lets you take full, deep breaths during challenging movement and postures that require focus and stability. You can use the structure of ujjayi breathing to help you in difficult poses and sequences.

The ujjayi breath is often called the ocean breath because of the soft whooshing sound you make by sending your inhales and exhales over the back of your throat. Learning to properly practice this breathing technique can be a challenge for some, so be patient with yourself.

Instruction

▤ Inhale through your nose, then open your mouth and exhale slowly through it while making a HA sound as if you were fogging up a mirror. Repeat a few times until you're comfortable making the HA sound on your exhale.

▤ Begin to inhale and exhale through your nose only, but keep the HA sound going on your exhales. This should create the soft whooshing sound of the ocean. Practice this until you feel comfortable making the sound with your mouth closed.

Skull Shining Breath (Kapalabhati)

This is the energizing breathing technique that I turn to for fast results. Practicing breathing in this way helps to wake up my mind in the morning, and I often practice this during the time my coffee is brewing. Here, the emphasis is mostly on the exhalation with strong contractions of your belly, creating exhales that push the air out of your lungs. Your inhales happen instinctually when the contraction of your belly finishes, triggering your lungs to suck air back into themselves.

Instruction

- Bring your focus to your belly, especially the mid- to low sections. Quickly and forcefully contract your muscles and exhale a big burst of air.

- Next, release the contraction all at once so that your lungs pull in your next inhale automatically. Practice this back and forth until you feel more adept at the contraction and quick release for the inhale to occur.

- You can practice this breathing technique for a couple minutes at a time, paying attention to the pace of your breathing. It's easy to accidentally increase the speed of your breath and find yourself going too fast for comfort. If that happens, just bring yourself back to your natural breath and start again at a slower pace. The more you practice kapalabhati breathing, the easier it gets to control the rhythm and pace of your breath. You've got this!

CONCLUSION

These warm-up stretches, movements, and breathing techniques are all great ways to prepare your body for the day, for your practice, or as a practice on their own. I encourage you to explore the range of seated positions, stretches, and breathing techniques in this chapter and beyond! There are so many ways to warm up your body and mind, and the more you practice them, the more integrated into your life they become. I have found immense help from these and other basic yogic actions and behaviors.

Learning to prioritize my comfort, whether it's about sitting on the floor or using props, has helped me to bring that empowered state into the rest of my life. I used to be afraid of bothering people with simple requests that would help me be more comfortable at restaurants, other public venues, and even friends' homes. My yoga practice has taught me to value my needs and to advocate for myself.

The gentle stretches, easy movement, and impactful pranayama have become parts of my daily routine. I count on them to help keep me feeling relaxed, connected, and inspired to move. I love that I no longer need to set alarms to remind me to stretch, stand up from my desk, take deeper breaths, or connect to my breath. My yoga practice has integrated into my life, and it takes care of me! I want this for you! Try the warm-up activities in this chapter, play around with finding comfortable ways to sit, and practice breathing in different ways. These all sound so simple, but their impact on your life can be incredible!

CHAPTER 4

SEATED AND KNEELING POSES

Some of my most practiced and most loved poses are the ones I do on the floor. I love seated poses because they're so accessible and easy to do even when I'm not feeling my best. Seated and kneeling poses offer a huge range of stretching, strengthening, and body connection. I often spend an entire home yoga practice on the floor and never stand up once. I teach some classes where we never stand up, and my students love them! I know the images of yoga postures we see online and in the media are usually standing or some kind of intense arm balance, but your practice doesn't have to look like that. You could never practice a single standing pose for the rest of your life and still have a strong and impactful yoga practice. It's not that I don't like standing poses, but I just love the freedom that seated and kneeling poses can bring to our practice.

A common misconception is that seated poses are easy. While many of them can be less intense to some people, there are plenty of seated and kneeling poses that provide a great challenge for those interested in pushing themselves. I appreciate the fact that we can make seated and kneeling poses as difficult as we want them to be. Creating accessible challenges for yourself is often simply a matter of using less support or altering your leg position in some way.

In this chapter, we'll dive into a number of seated and kneeling postures that I personally cherish and love to teach. I chose them for this book because they are my go-to poses for addressing the most common needs I often hear students discuss. These poses can help increase flexibility in all the major muscle groups. They can build strength in your core, arms, shoulders, back, and legs. It's a great group of poses to do all together as a single practice or to sprinkle into your personal practice or daily life whenever they're needed. I often find myself sitting down to do a couple of these at a time during my workday, especially when I've been sitting at the computer and feeling super tight all over.

This chapter includes a detailed explanation of all aspects of each featured pose:

- The benefits the pose can bring to your body and mind
- An alignment checklist, step-by-step instructions for how to get into the pose, and which sensations to look for in your body to know that you have the correct alignment
- Pose options to tailor the pose to work for your body as it is in that moment
- Ways to create accessible challenges for yourself, if you want to
- Any plus-size-specific tips that apply to the pose

Bound-Angle Pose (Baddha Konasana)

Ah, bound-angle pose—my favorite way to sit on the floor! This hip-opening posture can be practiced in a bunch of different ways to fit your body's needs in that moment. I love to come into the pose and then fold forward and hold for a few minutes to stretch the hips and lower back. I also really enjoy adding a little backbend for an opening restorative pose you can hold, with or without props, for support.

Bound-angle pose has a lot of benefits for your body, namely being a great stretch for your inner thighs, groin, hips, and lower back. I also really love this pose as a time to give my feet, ankles, knees, hips, and belly some extra love and attention. Since our focus is here already, I recommend using your hands to gently massage these parts to send a little gratitude their way.

Alignment Checklist

▥ Come to a seated position on the floor with a folded blanket underneath you if that helps you feel more comfortable. Bring the soles of your feet together and open your knees to each side to create an open space between them (see figure 4.1). Pull your heels in toward your pelvis as far as they comfortably can go while keeping your knees relaxed down toward the floor.

▥ Let your hands rest anywhere that is comfortable. Lengthen your spine, sitting as upright as possible. Let your hips be heavy and the crown of your head lift toward the ceiling.

▥ Stay here as long as you like, noticing the sensations in your pelvis, hips, knees, inner thighs, and anywhere else you feel activity. Experiment with holding the pose and taking deep breaths or practicing one of the pranayama techniques from chapter 3.

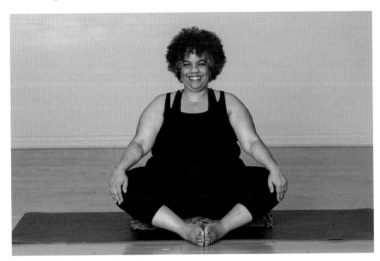

Figure 4.1 Bound-angle pose.

Pose Options

If sitting on the floor doesn't work for your body today, try this pose in bed following the same instructions. Or sit on a chair and bring your feet and ankles up to rest on another chair in front of you (see figure 4.2). Place a folded blanket under your feet if the chair seat is uncomfortable. Place blocks or rolled blankets under your knees if the unsupported version feels uncomfortable or unsafe.

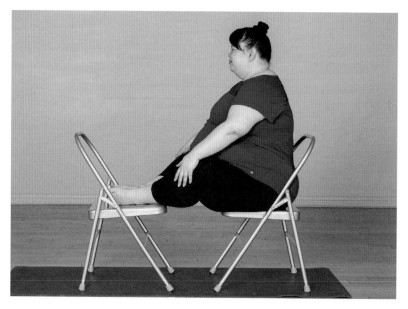

Figure 4.2   Bound-angle pose on a chair.

Accessible Challenges

■ Create an added challenge for yourself by pressing your knees down and holding, with or without the addition of raised arms.

■ Try folding forward and finding extra stretch in the hips and lower back.

Tips for Plus-Sized Bodies

Feel free to move your belly to make space and to make sitting upright on the floor more comfortable. Also, you can reach a couple fingers into the crease of your bent knee and move the skin upward if you feel compression behind the knees in this position.

Tabletop Pose (Bharmanasana)

While many consider this to be simply a transition pose between other postures or movements, I disagree! Tabletop pose is a great pose by itself, and it's a wonderful base to create accessible challenges for yourself. It can be tailored to your body's needs and capacity, bringing strengthening and stretching to you in balanced ways. Tabletop pose brings a gentle stretch to the arms, shoulders, wrists, hips, thighs, and spine. It's a great way to warm up the body for more intense poses and stretches to come.

Alignment Checklist

▥ From kneeling, bring your hands to the floor so that you are evenly distributing your weight through the hands and knees. Make sure your wrists are directly below your shoulders and that your knees are directly under your hips.

▥ Pull your belly in toward your spine so that your lower back doesn't arch. You want your spine to be parallel to the ceiling and in a long, straight line from the crown of your head to your tailbone (see figure 4.3).

▥ Spread your fingers apart and press through your fingertips to distribute your weight more evenly. Your gaze should be straight down at the floor so that the back of your neck is long.

▥ Hold here, breathing normally, for a few breaths. Notice what it feels like to hold here, to breathe in this position. You can move on to another pose or practice some of the accessible challenges that follow.

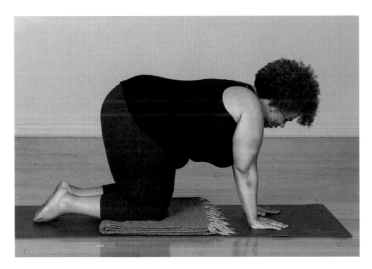

Figure 4.3 Tabletop pose.

Pose Options

▥ Add a folded blanket under your knees to protect them.

▥ A rolled blanket placed under your palms can help the wrists to be more comfortable in this position. If any amount of pressure on your wrists is too much, bring your forearms to blocks or a bolster instead.

▥ If kneeling is problematic, practice tabletop pose from standing with your hands or forearms on a chair seat.

Accessible Challenges

There are many ways to find accessible challenges in tabletop pose. Here is one of my favorites!

From tabletop, slide your left foot back until your leg is straight out behind you. Stay here or, if you choose, lift the leg straight up, keeping your knee and toes pointed down at the floor. Raise your right arm and reach out in front of you, arm parallel to the floor (see figure 4.4). You'll need to use your core to stabilize yourself and keep balanced. Make sure you keep your back flat and your gaze down. Hold the pose for a few breaths, and then release and repeat on the other side.

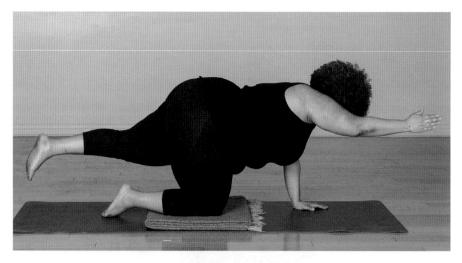

Figure 4.4   Tabletop pose with balance.

Cat–Cow Pose (Chakravakasana)

This duo is an amazingly accessible way to get your spine moving at any time, whether you're about to hit the mat or not. I find myself moving back and forth between the poses at my desk, while standing for long periods of time, in my car when I'm stuck in traffic, waiting in line at the grocery store, and, oh, yeah, also when I'm practicing yoga at home.

Cat–cow pose consists of two separate postures that are almost always practiced together because they combine to create a perfect spinal stretch. Give the kneeling version a try and see how it feels for your knees and wrists. If tabletop pose on your hands and knees is uncomfortable or feels unsafe, try practicing the seated version on the floor or in a chair. If you've only ever tried the kneeling version, be sure to experiment with the seated versions to experience the pose in new ways!

Cat–cow pose is a great spinal movement that is helpful in both grounding you to your body and your breath and in really focusing on the sensations of the chest, spine, and hips. The movement these poses create warms the body and increases flexibility in the spine while also opening the chest and shoulder blades.

Alignment Checklist

■ Come to your hands and knees with a folded blanket or kneepad under your knees if it's more comfortable. Check to make sure your knees are positioned right below your hips and your wrists are directly below your shoulders. Keep your head in a neutral position with your eyes looking straight down at the floor.

■ Inhale, pressing through your entire hands and fingers, lifting the tailbone and chest up toward the ceiling. Let your belly sink down toward the floor and your back arch into a C shape. Keep your head in line with your spine (see figure 4.5*a*).

■ On your exhale, reverse the position of your spine, rounding up toward the ceiling. Let your chin come down toward your chest and your tailbone tuck under (see figure 4.5*b*). You're making a C shape again here, just in the opposite direction.

■ Move back and forth between these two poses, experimenting with how it feels to be in each pose and how much of a C shape you can make each time. Stay here as long as you like, moving at the speed of your breath. Try to take the full length of your inhale to come into cow pose and the full length of your exhale to come into cat pose. Moving slowly, notice all the sensations you can find in your body as you practice these poses.

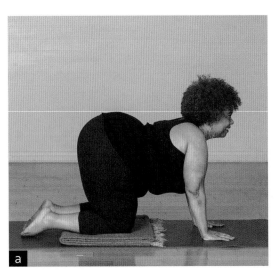 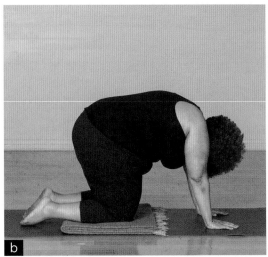

Figure 4.5 Cat–cow pose: *(a)* cow; *(b)* cat.

Pose Options

If kneeling doesn't feel comfortable or safe for your body, or if you're looking for a different way to experience this pose, try a seated version! You can sit on the floor or in a chair for this version. Sit in a way that your lower body is grounded and stable. If you're on the floor, sit in any comfortable position. If you're on a chair, be sure your feet can rest firmly on the floor or a supportive surface. Bring your hands to your knees or thighs and inhale, lifting your chest up and back. Your shoulders will probably move back, and your spine will begin to arch. Press through your hands to get a little help finding the arch of the back. Tilt your pelvis forward, letting your tailbone lift up, and make a C shape with your back (see figure 4.6*a*). On your exhale, press your hands into your legs to create leverage for help in rounding the spine. Tilt your pelvis backward and tuck your tailbone under while sending your shoulders forward. Round your back into a C shape and let your chin move toward your chest (see figure 4.6*b*). Move back and forth between these two poses, experimenting with how it feels to be in each pose and how much of a C shape you can make each time.

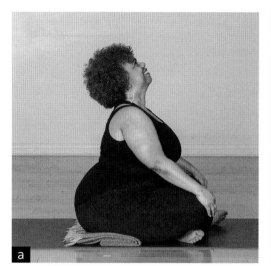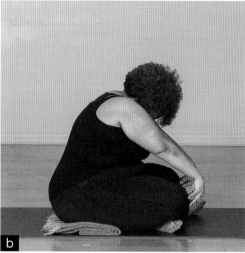

Figure 4.6 Seated cat–cow pose: *(a)* cow; *(b)* cat.

If the kneeling version works for you, except your wrists feel uncomfortable, try rolling a blanket a few times and placing it underneath your palms. This will tilt your hands at a different angle and can relieve pressure on your wrists.

Tips for Plus-Sized Bodies

If you practice the seated version on the floor, don't be afraid to move your belly to make sitting on the floor more comfortable. Slide it to the center or lift it up and place it on top of your thighs.

Simple Twist (Parivrtta Sukhasana)

I bet you already practice this one and don't even realize it! Simple twist is a basic pose we instinctively seek out when our backs and necks start bothering us. I love to practice simple twist at my desk, in the car, and on my mat as a way to get my spine gently moving. The benefits of this pose are impressive, with the twisting motion helping to relieve pain in the neck and back and also providing a stretch and opening for the chest and shoulders.

Alignment Checklist

▥ Begin in a comfortable seated position on the floor. Make sure your lower body is grounded and relaxed. Inhale, lifting your spine up long from the waist.

▥ Exhale and begin to twist to the left, moving first the lower spine and then the middle back and neck. Place the left hand on the floor or a block by your left hip (see figure 4.7). Your right hand can push off the right knee or cross over and pull from the left knee. Aim to keep your shoulders level, not letting the left shoulder dip low toward the floor. Hold for a few breaths. On an exhale, come back to center.

▥ Repeat to the right side to complete one full series. Twist once more in each direction, staying with your breath and taking your time to find the correct alignment.

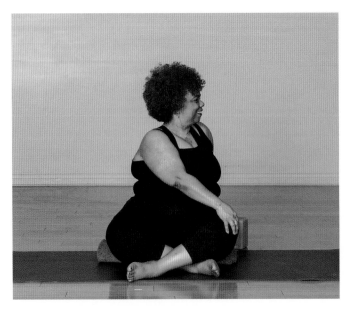

Figure 4.7 Seated simple twist pose.

Pose Options

Place blocks under your knees for support if that helps your lower body to relax. Practice the simple twist while seated on a chair, taking care to ground your feet on the floor or a sturdy surface.

Tips for Plus-Sized Bodies

▓ Move your belly to the center or up on top of your thighs if staying upright feels difficult.

▓ If it is difficult to reach across your belly, feel free to take a different option that works better for your body. For example, if you are twisting toward the left, let the front arm push off the right knee instead of reaching across the belly to pull from the left knee.

Camel Pose (Ustrasana)

There's something about a good backbend that feels really satisfying. Or maybe it's just me? Camel pose is one of those backbends that's so good at stretching not only the back but also the entire front of your body. What a multitasker! Camel is traditionally done from a kneeling position, but check the Pose Options section to see how to practice the pose from a chair. It's important to remember that the backbend here and in most other poses comes from lifting your chest, not from pressing your hips forward.

Alignment Checklist

- Come to a kneeling position with a folded blanket or kneepad under you. Make sure your knees are hip-width apart and your thighs are perpendicular to the floor. Press your shins and the tops of your feet firmly, but gently, into the floor to stabilize you and spread the weight of your body.

- Bring your hands to your back, palms resting below the dip of your lower back with your fingers pointing down.

- Inhale, lifting your chest straight up and letting your shoulders move back and down. Squeeze your elbows together any amount and lift your chin to keep your head in line with your spine (see figure 4.8).

- Hold here, noticing what the pose feels like in this position. Try not to press your hips forward to intensify the backbend. You can stay here for the duration of the pose.

- If you'd like, move your hands away from your body and reach the right hand toward the right foot and the left hand toward the left foot. If this works for you, hold here with your chest lifted. If reaching your feet doesn't work for you, tuck your toes under to raise your heels up a bit and see if that helps. If not, bring the hands back to your body and hold for a few breaths.

- Stay in this pose for a few breaths or as long as you feel comfortable. Come back to center by pressing off your body with your hands and gently lifting the head and torso up, leading with the head. If you feel dizzy, tuck your chin to your chest and hold there until the dizziness passes.

Pose Options

It's very likely that reaching your feet with your hands won't be in the cards for you. Take heart! Many seasoned yogis struggle to reach their feet, so don't feel bad. Also, don't ever feel bad for making a yoga pose your own. You can do that here by tucking the toes under to lift the feet higher as I described earlier. Also, here are other options to make the pose work for you in different ways depending on what your body needs:

- Try placing blocks just outside each heel, at their highest height, and bring your hands to the blocks.
- Place a bolster or stack of folded blankets directly on your calves or feet, and bring your hands to the top (see figure 4.9). You can stack support as high as you need to be able to reach.
- You can always bring the whole thing up to a chair! Sit toward the front of the chair seat and follow the previously mentioned directions. Instead of bringing your hands to your feet, reach for the chair back or chair seat.

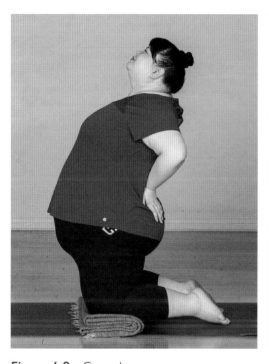

Figure 4.8 Camel pose.

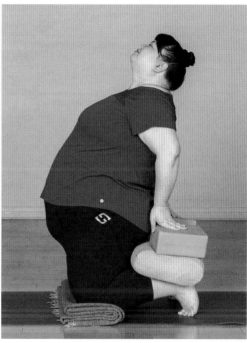

Figure 4.9 Camel pose with bolster and blocks on legs.

Accessible Challenges

Try bumping up the challenge by bringing your thighs, calves, and feet closer together.

Tips for Plus-Sized Bodies

If you feel unstable, check in with your thighs. Sometimes pressing them too close together can push you out of alignment and cause you to feel unstable or uncomfortable. Step your knees farther apart and see how that feels.

Gate Pose (Parighasana)

Oh, this one is so fun! Gate pose is a cool way to explore a side stretch, balance work, and even some strengthening all at the same time. You can stretch your torso and spine, activate your core with balance work, and build strength all over with some pose options to add accessible challenges. Try practicing gate pose in different ways to feel the range of sensations possible. Don't forget to use props to find support where it's needed.

Alignment Checklist

- From kneeling, bring your right leg out to the side and turn the knee and toes up to the ceiling, rotating from the hip. Press your right heel down firmly, slightly turning toes in if that's more comfortable. Your left knee should be directly under your left hip, and your torso should be lifted tall.

- Inhale and lift your torso. Exhale, coming into a side-bend to the right. Bring your right hand to your right thigh or calf, not your knee. Reach your left arm up and over, stretching the left side of your body as much as possible. Keep your torso and hips turned to the front, not twisting toward your straight leg. Hold for a few breaths and continue to stretch your left side (see figure 4.10*a*).

- Inhale and bring yourself back to upright. Keeping your right leg in position, exhale while side-bending to the left, and bring your left hand to the floor or a block. Find your stability here and then sweep your right arm up and over, stretching long through the right side of your body. Think of making a very straight line from right fingertips to right toes (see figure 4.10*b*).

- Stay here for a few breaths and then come up on an inhale. Switch legs and repeat on the left side.

Pose Options

If the floor feels far away, place a block under your hand (see figure 4.11*a*).

Gate pose can also be done while seated on a chair. Sit toward the front of your chair so that most of your thighs are off the seat. Let your left ankle line up directly under your left knee. Send your right leg out to the side exactly as the earlier instructions explain (see figure 4.11*b*). The pose can be completed in the same way as the kneeling version with the exception of hand placement. For stability, hold the chair seat when side-bending over the bent leg.

Accessible Challenges

Try lifting the straight leg once you come into the second phase of the pose. Stabilize your hand on the floor or a block and sweep the opposite arm up and over so that your body is super long. Then play with raising the straight leg as high as it feels like a challenge for you today.

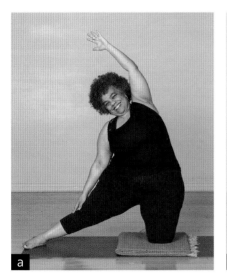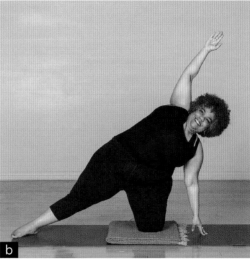

Figure 4.10 Kneeling gate pose: *(a)* stretch toward extended right leg; *(b)* stretch to left side.

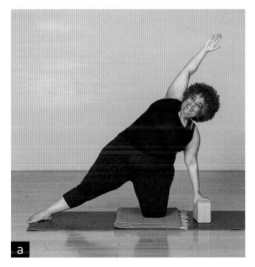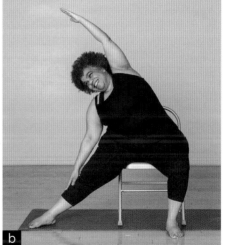

Figure 4.11 Gate pose: *(a)* kneeling with block under hand and blanket under knee; *(b)* in a chair.

Head-to-Knee Pose (Janu Sirsasana)

This seated pose is a wonderful way to open the chest and stretch the back of the legs and lower back. If you find stretching forward over both straight legs to be painful, this pose can be a helpful alternative. By bending one of your legs, you can find a great stretch for the other without a struggle. I love to teach this posture with a strap, which allows you to get a sustained stretch without straining your arms and shoulders or bringing yourself out of alignment.

Alignment Checklist

■ Sit on the floor with your legs straight out to the front. Bend one knee, open it out to the side, and bring the sole of your foot to rest against the inside of the straight leg.

■ Loop the middle of your strap around the ball of the straight leg's foot. Lift up through your torso and bring your shoulders slightly back and down. Hold one end of the strap with each hand, and walk your hands forward as far as you can while keeping your spine very straight and long.

■ Hinge forward from the hips as you lower your torso toward your straight leg, keeping your back straight and chest lifted (see figure 4.12). Lead with your chest, not your shoulders or head, to keep in alignment. Hold here for a few breaths, allowing your body to relax into the stretch. Then inhale yourself up to center and switch sides.

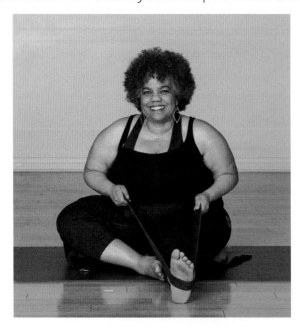

Figure 4.12   Head-to-knee pose seated on a folded blanket.

Pose Options

This pose can be done from a chair by placing your legs up on a second chair in front of you (see figure 4.13). The instructions are the same!

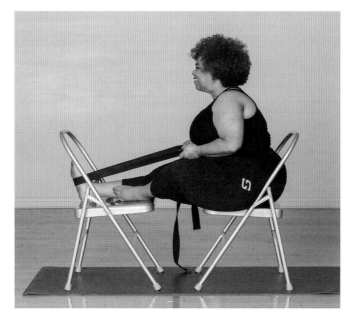

Figure 4.13   Head-to-knee pose seated on a chair with legs up on a second chair.

Accessible Challenges

Experiment without using a strap!

Tips for Plus-Sized Bodies

This may be a helpful time to try lifting your belly up and placing it on top of your thighs. This creates space where your hips meet your thighs and can help you find a deeper hinge forward.

Wide-Leg Forward-Fold Pose (Upavistha Konasana)

A wonderful way to stretch the backs of your legs and inner thighs, wide-leg forward-fold is also great for strengthening your back and improving your posture. There's a lot of room for customization here, with varying arm positions, hold times, and prop options to provide support. This pose is almost always in my home practice and classes. It's a classic crowd-pleaser!

Alignment Checklist

- Sit on the floor and open the legs into a wide V. Make little adjustments as needed to bring the legs wider or to distribute weight more evenly between left and right sides of the body. Rotate your legs from the hips so that your knees and toes point straight up toward the ceiling. Add a soft flex of your feet to engage the muscles up the backs of your legs.

- Inhale, sweeping the arms overhead, and then exhale as you hinge from the hips and fold forward with a straight back. Lead with your chest, not your shoulders. You want to keep your spine long!

- Come forward as far as you need to in order to feel a stretch up the backs of your legs. Rest your hands on your feet, the floor, blocks, or another support and keep your back straight (see figure 4.14). Stay for a few breaths or longer if it's comfortable to do so. When you're ready, inhale and roll up slowly to center.

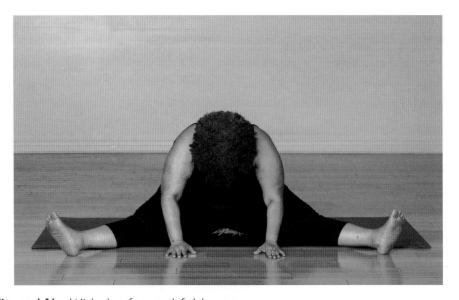

Figure 4.14 Wide-leg forward-fold pose.

Pose Options

■ Bring your hands or forearms to blocks, a bolster, or a stack of blankets to find support and be able to keep your spine straight.

■ Practice wide-leg forward-fold from seated on a chair with each leg resting on another chair. This is a great way to practice when coming to the floor is not possible or desirable.

Accessible Challenges

An easy way to find extra challenge here is to simply lengthen the duration of your hold, bring yourself down lower, or add more flex to your feet.

Tips for Plus-Sized Bodies

You may find it helpful to slide your belly toward the open space between your legs in order to come down lower.

Low-Lunge Pose (Anjaneyasana)

Low-lunge is an excellent way to stretch and strengthen your legs, knees, and ankles. Practicing this pose helps with balance and stretching the hip flexors, which can improve your posture over time. Commonly practiced from a kneeling position, check the Pose Options section for information on how to perform it while standing.

Alignment Checklist

■ From a kneeling position, bring your right foot forward to rest the sole of the foot on the mat with your heel directly under your right knee. Think of a classic marriage proposal position: down on one knee. Make sure the top of your left foot is on the floor so that the toes are not tucked under.

■ Press your hips forward, finding a stretch in the groin area and down the front of your left thigh. Let your weight shift forward so that the top of your left knee makes contact with the floor (see figure 4.15). If you don't feel the stretch in your left thigh, play with scooting your right foot forward a little and then pressing your hips forward again. Be sure to lead with your hips, not your chest.

■ You can place your hands on blocks on either side of your right knee, bring your hands to rest on your right knee, or lift your arms up toward the ceiling. Hold the pose for a few breaths or as long as you're comfortable. Then either pull the right leg back down into a kneeling position or transition to half-monkey pose (page 82) and then switch sides.

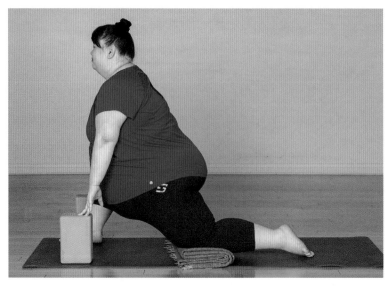

Figure 4.15   Low-lunge pose.

Pose Options

Placing padding under your knees and using blocks under your hands make this pose more comfortable for most practitioners.

If kneeling is not possible, or you'd like to experience the pose in a new way, try the standing version with a chair! Stand about a leg's distance away from a sturdy chair, facing the chair seat. Bring your leg up and forward to rest your left foot firmly on the center of the seat. Press your hips forward, finding a stretch in the groin area and down the front of your right thigh (see figure 4.16). If you don't feel the stretch in your right thigh, play with scooting your right foot backward a little and then pressing your hips forward again. Be sure to lead with your hips, not your chest. Hold the pose for a few breaths or as long as you're comfortable. Then either pull the left leg back down into a standing position or transition to half-monkey pose (page 82) and then switch sides.

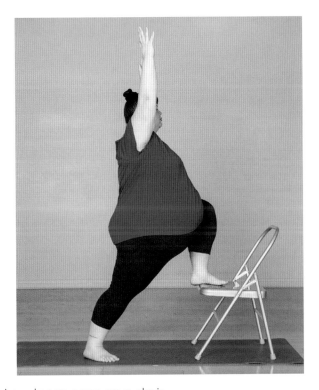

Figure 4.16 Low-lunge pose on a chair.

Accessible Challenges

■ Once in your lunge, add a backbend to increase the difficulty level.

■ Try increasing the distance between your front foot and the supporting knee. The greater the distance between the two, the lower you'll need to lunge.

Half-Monkey Pose (Ardha Hanumanasana)

Usually practiced in conjunction with low-lunge pose, half-monkey is a wonderful hamstrings stretch that can prepare the body for the rest of your practice and help prevent lower-body injury. If kneeling is uncomfortable, check the Pose Options section for a standing version.

Alignment Checklist

■ From a kneeling position, bring your left foot forward to rest the sole of the foot on the mat with your heel directly under your left knee. Again, think of a classic marriage proposal position: down on one knee. Make sure the top of your right foot is on the floor so that the toes are not tucked under.

■ Slide your left leg into a straight position, coming out directly to the front. Flex your foot, with only your heel connected to the ground, with knee and toes facing upward to the ceiling.

■ Bring your hands to two blocks on either side of your left leg, and hinge forward to bring your torso down toward your left leg (see figure 4.17). Lower yourself down until you feel a stretch in the back of the leg.

■ Stay here for a few breaths and then, pressing through your hands, bend the left knee and return it to the starting position. You can switch legs and repeat on the other side or transition to low-lunge on the right side and then follow with half-monkey pose.

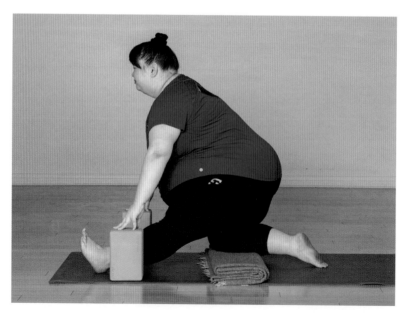

Figure 4.17   Half-monkey pose.

Pose Options

If kneeling is not possible, try the standing version. Stand about a leg's distance away from a sturdy chair, facing the chair seat. Bring your leg up and forward to rest your right foot firmly on the center of the seat. Slide your right leg into a straight position, coming out directly to the front. Flex your foot, with only your heel connected to the seat, with knee and toes facing upward to the ceiling. Bring your hands to rest on your right thigh or shin, not your knee, and hinge forward to bring your torso down toward your right leg (see figure 4.18). Lower yourself down until you feel a stretch in the back of the leg. Stay here for a few breaths and then release your hands, bringing your torso up to center. You can switch legs and repeat on the other side or transition to low-lunge on the left side and then follow with half-monkey pose.

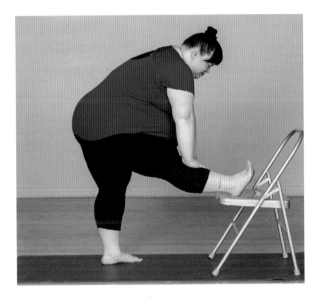

Figure 4.18 Half-monkey pose on a chair.

Accessible Challenges

■ Consider working toward monkey pose, a full split. You begin in the same way as half-monkey and then slide your back leg out straight behind you with your pelvis near the floor. If you attempt this, put a bolster or folded blankets under your hips to provide some support.

■ Not ready for full monkey? Try rotating your blocks to a lower height or sliding the back of your knee back a little farther to bring your pelvis lower.

Z-Sit Pose (Pinwheel)

Z-sit is a great pose to loosen up tight hips and glutes so they're ready for the rest of your practice. This gentle hip stretch lets you work on internal and external hip rotation at the same time. Also sometimes called pinwheel pose, this seated posture can be done with different torso and arm positions to change the sensations you feel. However, at its core, z-sit is a wonderful resting stretch that will bring lots of benefits without moving an inch!

Alignment Checklist

▥ Sit on the floor with the soles of the feet together and knees open to the sides, as you would set up for a bound-angle pose.

▥ Lean to the right, bringing your right hand to the floor for support. Pick up your left leg and bend it behind you to make a pinwheel shape with your legs. Slide your right foot over to the left to bring your right knee out directly from the hip (see figure 4.19). Flex both feet.

▥ Sit up tall and lifted from your hips and hold for a few breaths before switching sides.

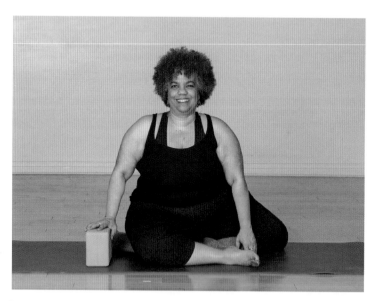

Figure 4.19 Z-sit pose.

Pose Options

▦ Sit up on a folded blanket to raise your hips to make sitting on the floor more comfortable.

▦ If staying upright feels difficult, place a block or other supportive prop under your hand to bring the floor up to you and give you something from which to push off.

Accessible Challenges

Try different torso and arm positions while holding the pose to increase the stretch:

▦ Lift the arms up and then forward-fold over the front leg, holding for as long as feels comfortable. Be sure to stay centered over the hips and not off to the side.

▦ Add a side-bend, sweeping the arm on the front-leg side up and over to the opposite side and holding for a few breaths. Switch arms each time you switch legs.

▦ Experiment with reaching your torso and arms in different directions. Find new sensations and stretches!

Tips for Plus-Sized Bodies

You can reach a couple fingers into the crease of your bent knee and move the flesh upward if you feel compression behind the knees in this position.

Plank Pose (Kumbhakasana)

Plank is one of those poses that gets a bad rap because it's very challenging for a lot of people. There's much to be gained by practicing it though, and I have some great ways to make this pose more accessible. Usually, we save the most supported versions for the Pose Options section, but for plank, I think it's great to start with a lot of support. You can always remove some if you want to hold more of your weight. Read on for lots of ideas on how to make this total-body strengthening pose work for you!

Alignment Checklist

■ Place a bolster or a stack of folded blankets up the length of your mat. This will be the support for your torso. Come to hands and knees, or tabletop pose, with the support directly under your torso. Stretch one leg back until it's straight, and then tuck your toes under. Repeat with the other leg and adjust your hips down until your body is close to a straight line from the crown of your head to the heels (see figure 4.20).

■ Check in with your support to make sure it's tall enough to hold you up. You may need to adjust the height to rise up to meet your torso. Once it's firmly holding you, play with pressing through your arms and legs to use the amount of support that feels right to you. Some days you might want more support, and some days less will feel right.

■ Hold here for a few breaths or as long as you are comfortable. Come down to rest before repeating or transitioning to another pose.

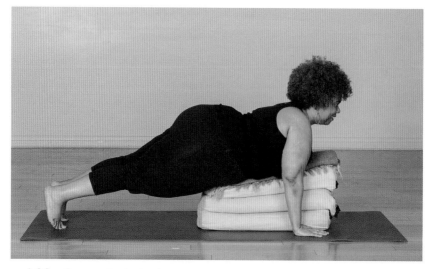

Figure 4.20 Supported plank pose.

Pose Options

If you decide to use less support under your torso, you might still want a little something to assist you. Try looping and securing a strap around your arms, just above your elbows. As you come into plank, press your arms out against this strap. The tension of the strap will help take some of the weight of your body as you hold plank.

If the floor version doesn't feel right, or you want to experience the pose in new ways, try practicing plank pose on a chair or the wall. To practice on a chair, stand in front of a chair that won't slide. Fold forward and bring your hands to the chair seat. Stay down in the folded position and find a stable grip; holding on to each side of the chair seat always feels stable to me. Walk your feet back a few steps and then lift your heels and press forward into your hands. Press your hips forward until your body comes into a straight line (see figure 4.21) and hold for a few breaths. When you're ready, bring your heels down and walk your feet back toward the chair, then roll up slowly.

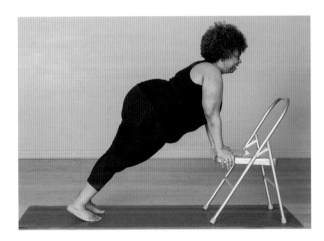

Figure 4.21 Plank pose on a chair.

To practice on the wall, start in a standing position facing the wall and bring your hands to it at about shoulder height. Walk your feet back a few steps and then lift your heels and press forward into your hands. Press your hips forward until your body comes into a straight line and hold for a few breaths. You may need to experiment with how far back you need to step in order to find a plank that works for you. The farther away you step your feet, the lower your hands need to move down the wall. When you're ready, bring your heels down and walk your feet back toward the wall, then roll up slowly.

Accessible Challenges

- ■ In any version of plank, try lifting a leg to add some challenge.
- ■ You can play with moving from the wall to the chair and then down to the floor to progressively increase the amount of weight you're holding with your arms.

CONCLUSION

You did it! You made it through our first chapter of poses like a champ! What did you think? Were there poses that appealed to you immediately or some that seemed scary or unpleasant? It's nice to take stock of how you're feeling as you learn about the different types of postures. Honor whatever thoughts and emotions are coming up for you right now. What does your body need? Are you ready to hit the mat and excited to try out some of these poses? Or are you feeling overwhelmed and needing to step back for a bit and come back to it later? There's no wrong way to be feeling right now. Mindfully noticing your sensations, thoughts, energy, and mood is part of practicing yoga.

We've taken a look at some seated and kneeling postures that you can experiment with and see what works for your body. Remember that your practice can look and feel any way you'd like it to. You could practice only these poses for the rest of your life and still experience a rich, personal practice. I hope you explore these poses and experiment with finding the perfect way to soothe tired muscles, raise your energy level, build strength, and work out the kinks from sitting or standing too long.

My goal with this chapter is to show you that there are tons of ways to find accessible options and challenges from the floor or a chair, and that it can be really fun to invent new ways to stretch, strengthen, and connect with your body. There are floor-based sequences in chapters 9 and 10, so you can try out these postures and see how it feels to practice without standing up. I love allowing myself to spend the entire practice on the floor without coming up to standing at all! Or you can mix them with standing poses and see how that feels for your body. The wonderful thing about a yoga practice is that you get to call the shots because you're the boss!

The next chapter introduces standing poses that will increase your ability to practice and provide lots of options. These seated and kneeling postures are perfect accompaniments to the standing poses as they prepare your body for what comes after you stand up. Take your time prepping with the poses we've just covered and then you'll be ready to move on if you're feeling like it. Many of the seated and kneeling poses are also excellent for after you practice the standing postures, so with these two chapters combined you're set to get creative and start to practice yoga. Are you excited? Are you scared? Are you feeling a little of both? That's totally normal and to be expected. Take a deep breath, get a drink of water, and remind yourself that you are the boss and you've got this!

CHAPTER 5

STANDING POSES

The world of standing yoga poses is vast, but at the core of all of them is a common principle: We root down to rise. From standing, we can anchor ourselves to the floor and find length, strength, and freedom in postures that bring attention to every part of the body. Whether you're looking for flexibility, strength building, or embodiment, I know these standing poses will provide what you seek! I hope you find the exploration of these poses as interesting and exciting as I do. Remember, the pose is a starting point! Learn the alignment and benefits available, and then jump off and explore all the many ways to make these poses your own. There are countless pose options and accessible challenges for you to experiment with to find what works for your body.

Throughout this chapter, you'll continue to see options to try if you'd like to experience poses in new ways or find greater accessibility. While this chapter is about standing poses, there are plenty of ways to use a chair for partial or full support. Try some of these options even if you don't feel you need them. You might find a new way of approaching a pose that shifts your perspective or provides a new benefit! It's important to think of props and options as interesting and helpful benefits instead of as consolation prizes. The culture of judgment does us no good when it comes to the amazing advantages that props and pose options can bring to your practice.

In this chapter, you'll learn about standing poses, taking time to understand how and why to enrich your practice with these classics. I've chosen these postures because they're all great on their own, and, put together, they can build amazing sequences to help you reach any goals you have. Depending on what you're working toward, these poses can help you feel grounded, work on your balance, build strength, improve your flexibility, and increase your stamina. You can tailor your practice to bring gentle movement, grounding, and breath work into your morning or before going to bed. Or you can follow a sequence to build energy and get your body moving and warm before tackling the rest of the day. Standing poses are a strong part of a yoga practice and can be endlessly adapted to fit your exact needs.

Each pose in the chapter has its own section with a detailed explanation of all aspects of the pose, including the following:

- The benefits the pose can bring to your body and mind
- An alignment checklist, step-by-step instructions for how to get into the pose, and what sensations to look for in your body to know that you have the correct alignment
- Pose options to tailor the pose to work for your body as it is in that moment
- Ways to create accessible challenges for yourself, if you want to
- Any plus-size-specific tips that apply to the pose

Mountain Pose (Tadasana)

Mountain pose is my most practiced asana. It is a wonderful pose on its own and also a perfect transition posture during a standing practice. Whether I'm teaching or practicing on my own, I use mountain as a recalibrating pose between every standing posture. It's also an amazing way to practice off the mat! Try coming into mountain pose while waiting in line at the grocery store or whenever you're standing for a long time. The alignment of the pose is a great way to protect your body when standing still. You can keep yourself from slumping over, shifting weight side to side constantly, and getting stiff knees. Plus, it's a great way to ground yourself and stay connected to your body throughout your day.

Mountain pose is very grounding and stabilizing, just as a real mountain is. The alignment of the pose is very important, and you should pay close attention to the details throughout your body. If you're new to the alignment of mountain, it may seem like a lot to remember. Don't worry! The more you practice it, the easier it will be to name the elements of the Alignment Checklist. Since we return to mountain pose so often, you'll get lots of practice!

Alignment Checklist

- Stand with your feet a comfortable distance apart. They should be about hip-distance apart, but take care to measure your hip distance by the bones and not the flesh of your body. You're looking for your legs to come straight down from the hip joints and not out at a diagonal.

- Press down evenly on all four sides of your feet. Check in with the balls of your feet, heels, outer edges, and inner edges. You want to feel each side press down firmly into the floor. This is the foundation of the pose, so start strong by rooting down into the floor.

- Pull up tall through your legs, but be careful not to lock your knees. Soften, or very slightly bend, your knees throughout the duration of mountain pose. The bend may be so slight that it's imperceptible to others, but you should feel that your knees are not locked.

- Bring your pelvis to neutral so that your tailbone is not tilted to the front or the back. It may be helpful to tilt your pelvis forward and backward a few times to feel where neutral is.

- Lengthen your torso up from the waist, lifting your spine tall while sending shoulders down and back. Think of opening across your collarbone and creating a tiny pinch in between your shoulder blades.

▥ Rotate your arms from the shoulders so that the insides of your arms face forward. Hold them in a low V shape. Make sure your shoulders aren't crowding up near your ears; you can actively press them down toward the ground.

▥ Finally, tuck your chin very slightly down toward your chest to lengthen the back of your neck (see figure 5.1). Think of raising the crown of your head up toward the ceiling.

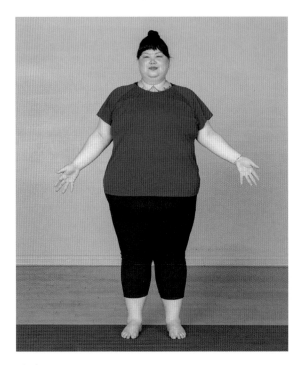

Figure 5.1 Mountain pose.

Pose Options

Mountain pose can absolutely be practiced from seated on a chair (see figure 5.2):

▥ Sit on a chair with your feet firmly planted on the ground, ankles directly below your knees. If your feet do not easily rest on the ground, bring the floor up to them by placing a block or firm bolster underfoot.

▥ Press down evenly through your feet and hips and lift your torso up from the waist. All the other instructions are exactly the same as the standing version!

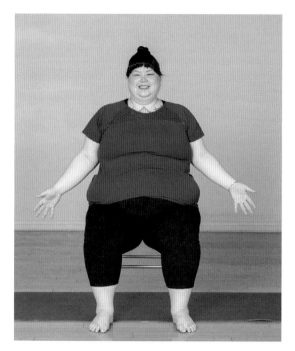

Figure 5.2   Mountain pose on a chair.

Accessible Challenges

You can find extra challenge by engaging all your muscles while holding mountain pose. Imagine you are standing on a piece of paper. Press your feet down into the floor and energetically out to each side as if you could rip the paper in half. Feel your outer thighs engage and add your inner thighs as well. Hold your core tight, engage the muscles in your chest and arms, and breathe with intention. Hold this active version of mountain pose as long as feels like a challenge for you.

Tips for Plus-Sized Bodies

If bringing your feet very close together causes discomfort in your thighs or where your knees touch, step a little farther apart until you feel more comfortable.

Forward-Fold Pose (Uttanasana)

Forward-fold is one of those poses that can feel intense or gentle depending on how your body is feeling that day. I think that's cool because it becomes a barometer to help you gauge what your body needs at any given time. What's great about forward-fold is that because you can do it in so many ways, there is always an option to fit your needs.

A lot of times, I hear people say that they're not flexible enough to do yoga and, usually, they're thinking of trying to touch their toes. I hope you hear me when I say that you don't have to touch your toes! Sure, your goal might be to touch your toes, but forward-fold is about so much more than that. The benefits you can experience include stretching the legs and back, of course. However, forward-fold also allows you to get the calming effects of an inversion and also may help with headaches and fatigue.

Alignment Checklist

■ Begin by coming into mountain pose. Inhale and raise your arms to the ceiling. Exhale, bend your knees a little, and hinge at the waist to fold forward. Keep your spine long and straight as you come down and bring your hands to two blocks. Start with your blocks on the tallest side at first. You can always adjust them later.

■ With hands on the blocks for support, you can straighten your legs. Allow yourself to hold weight with your hands on the blocks (see figure 5.3). Find the straightest leg position you can and then adjust your blocks to a height that gives you support and allows your arms to straighten.

■ Relax your neck so your head can hang down. Hold here for a few breaths and then soften your knees and gently come up to standing. Repeat as many times as you like.

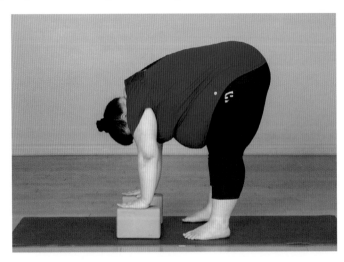

Figure 5.3　Forward-fold with blocks.

Pose Options

Try bringing your hands or forearms to a chair seat for a taller support.

Accessible Challenges

- Adjust your blocks to a lower height or try to bring your hands to the floor.
- Place a folded blanket underneath your toes or balls of the feet and fold forward. Notice how this feels in your legs.

Tips for Plus-Sized Bodies

- Step your feet a little wider apart to make space for your belly.
- Move your belly to the center to find a little more release in your back and bring your hands farther down toward the floor.

Downward-Facing Dog Pose (Adho Mukha Svanasana)

When I first started yoga, I loathed downward-facing dog! Instructors would call it a resting pose and have us hold it for a long time. I was miserable and hated when it was taught, and, unfortunately, it's a really popular pose that is included in almost every class. I felt shame that downward-facing dog wasn't a resting pose for me. I thought that my body was the problem and that it just couldn't do it right. I've found that this is a very common belief among larger-bodied yogis. I'm here to tell you that it's not true. Your body is not the problem! Downward-facing dog is not a resting pose if you're not taught ways to make it work for you.

My relationship with the posture changed once I learned that I could use props to make the pose more accessible for my body. Now that I know what to do, I can bring myself into proper alignment and experience the benefits of the pose instead of just struggling to be there. I'm really excited to share these tips with you. I hope I can spare you the pain of struggling through when you could be enjoying the pose!

Practicing downward-facing dog has some real benefits. It can be a gentle, calming inversion and stretch for your hamstrings, hips, back, and shoulders. The pose is also a nice way to build strength and find ways to transition between other poses, both standing and seated.

Alignment Checklist

- From mountain pose, inhale and lift your arms to stretch your body long. Exhale and forward-fold with soft knees, bringing your hands to two blocks on the ground in front of you.
- Holding the blocks in your hands, walk your hands forward a few feet.
- Shift your weight back into your legs, straightening them as much as feels comfortable (see figure 5.4). You want to hold most of your weight in your legs, not your hands. Think of pressing your thighs straight back to the wall behind you. Try lifting your hips up and back.
- You can adjust how the pose feels by walking your hands farther away and experimenting with straightening your legs more. Hold here for a few breaths and then bend your knees and walk your hands and feet toward each other. Come to forward-fold and then gently roll up to standing.

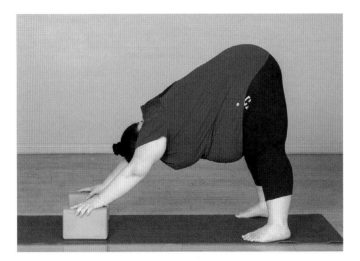

Figure 5.4   Downward-facing dog pose.

Pose Options

- You can change the height of your blocks to find more or less support.
- Try the chair version of the pose (see figure 5.5)! Stand in front of a sturdy chair on a nonslip surface. Forward-fold with soft knees, bringing your hands to the chair seat. Step your feet back until your arms are stretched long but your hands still rest easily on the chair seat. From here, the instructions are the same!

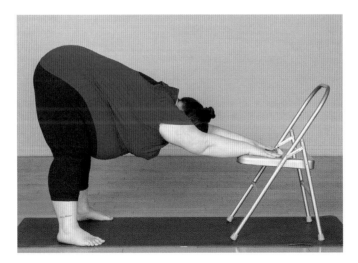

Figure 5.5   Downward-facing dog pose on a chair.

Accessible Challenges

▥ Try bringing a little more weight into your hands and lifting a leg up as high as is comfortable. Be sure to do both sides.

▥ Play with some dynamic movement and build upper-body strength by shifting forward into plank pose and then back into downward-facing dog. You can do this with your hands on blocks or a chair.

Tips for Plus-Sized Bodies

▥ Try stepping your feet wider apart to make space for your belly.

▥ If your breasts shift down to press on your throat, consider wrapping a looped strap around you to hold them in place. Some companies sell stretchy bands for this purpose!

Tree Pose (Vrksasana)

Tree pose is probably one of the most universally known yoga postures. Most of us knew what it was before we ever tried yoga, and yet there are so many myths about it. I'm excited to dig into the pose a little more and help to clear up some of the misconceptions. Tree pose does not need to be practiced with a foot to the thigh, with the bent knee facing straight out to the side, or even while standing!

Tree pose is an excellent way to build strength in your whole body, work on your balance, and help you feel centered and grounded. There are many different ways to experience tree pose, but the benefits never change. Whether you practice lying down on the floor or standing with support—or completely without—you can gain so much from adding tree to your practice. Be sure to check the Pose Options section to learn about different ways you can experience tree pose and make it work for your body.

Alignment Checklist

- Begin in mountain pose. Shift your weight onto your left foot so that only the toes of your right foot touch the floor. Find your balance here before moving on.

- Open your right leg out to the side, moving from the hip. Your right knee and toes should move from facing forward to facing out to the right at a diagonal. Slide your right foot over toward the left leg until your right heel touches your left ankle.

- Stay here in kickstand, with your right toes on the floor and your right heel on your left ankle, or slide your right foot up onto your left calf or thigh (see figure 5.6).

- It can be helpful when balancing to pick a spot on the wall or in the room to fix your gaze on. Choose something that's not moving and hold it in sight to ground your focus.

- Press your right foot into the inside of your left ankle or leg and your left ankle or leg into your right foot to help stabilize yourself.

- Keep your hips facing straight ahead. This is often called *squaring your hips*. Try to open your right leg, from the hip, as much as you can but don't force it.

- Hold your core muscles tight and stand tall and straight. If you'd like, you can bring your arms up into a high V or palms together at your chest for anjali mudra, the classic position also known as prayer hands. This hand position can be helpful in stabilizing you as you work on your balance.

- Hold here for a few breaths or as long as feels good to you. Repeat, balancing on the right leg.

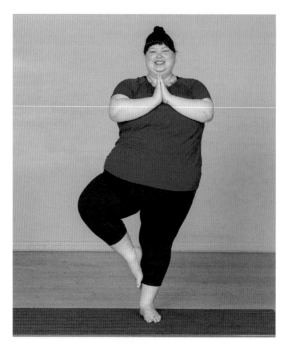

Figure 5.6 Tree pose with prayer hands.

Pose Options

■ Try tree pose with your back touching a wall for support. Stand in front of the wall so that your body is only lightly touching (see figure 5.7*a*). Be sure not to lean on the wall. Practice the pose according to the instructions above, but with the slight connection to the wall. Even a little support can bring a lot of stabilization.

■ Give the bent leg some support by resting your foot on a block placed directly next to your supporting leg (see figure 5.7*b*).

■ Work on learning the alignment of tree pose by practicing it on the floor. Lie on your back and come to mountain pose. It's the same as the standing version, only your support is under your back and legs instead of just under your feet. Follow the instructions for tree pose (see figure 5.7*c*) and notice what your spine and hips feel as you hold the posture.

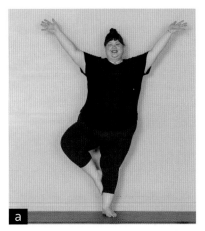

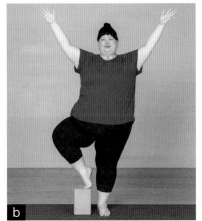
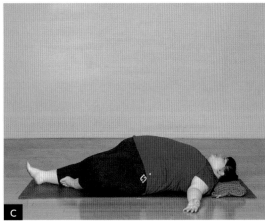

Figure 5.7 Tree pose options: *(a)* against a wall; *(b)* with a block; *(c)* on the floor.

Accessible Challenges

■ Hold tree pose and bring your arms up into a high V. Slowly wave them side to side and follow your hands with your gaze.

■ Try closing your eyes. Notice how closing your eyes affects your balance.

Tips for Plus-Sized Bodies

If you find compression in the area where your bent leg's calf and thigh come together near the back of the knee, you can try to create a little more spaciousness there. Imagine your right leg is feeling this compression. Insert your right index and middle fingers between the calf and thigh near the back of your knee. Gently, but firmly, push up into the thigh and bring the skin forward. For some, this is a helpful way to create a little extra room when the leg is bent in poses such as tree and bound-angle.

Chair Pose (Utkatasana)

This is a fun pose to try when you want to warm up quickly and prepare your body for the rest of your practice. With lots of options available to customize it for your body, chair pose is an accessible posture that fits into many sequences. Known mostly as a standing pose, it also works easily from seated on a chair.

The benefits of chair pose are varied and vast! It is a wonderful way to work on strengthening your feet, ankles, thighs, calves, core, and back. You can also add a balance or twisting element to it to level up and multitask. Try different arm positions to see what works best for your body and your changing needs.

Alignment Checklist

■ Begin in mountain pose. Inhale and bend your knees, bringing your tailbone down as if you were going to sit on a chair. Depending on how low you choose to squat, your thighs may come parallel to the floor.

■ Exhale and raise your arms overhead with palms facing in. Keep your chest lifted and your torso upright. Your gaze should be straight ahead.

■ Bring your shoulders back and down, lifting your chest and making space between your shoulders and ears (see figure 5.8).

■ Hold here for a few breaths or as long as feels comfortable. Come out of the pose by inhaling and straightening the knees. Lift through your arms and then exhale and come back into mountain pose.

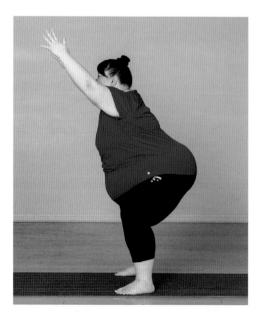

Figure 5.8 Chair pose.

Pose Options

Try a supported version of chair pose from a seated position. Sit on a chair in mountain pose. Inhale, raise your arms overheard with palms facing in, and press firmly into your feet as if you were going to stand up (see figure 5.9). You'll feel the muscles in your thighs, core, and buttocks engage and help you lift slightly off the seat. Your body will still be connected to the chair, but your muscles will be working to hold you up a little. You can decide how much you want to lift. Exhale and hold for a few breaths before returning to a seated position.

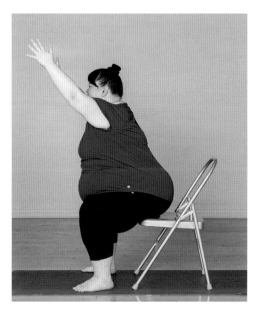

Figure 5.9   Chair pose from a chair.

Accessible Challenges

■ Level up the work your thighs are doing by squeezing a block between them as you hold the posture (see figure 5.10*a*).

■ Add a balance element by coming into the pose and then raising up onto the balls of your feet and toes (see figure 5.10*b*). Hold as long as it feels like a personal challenge for you.

■ Add a twisting element. Come into chair pose and then inhale and bring the palms together at the chest while lifting your spine tall. Exhale and twist your torso to the right, keeping your hips and knees to the front (see figure 5.10*c*). Hold as long as you like and then exhale back to the center. Repeat to the left side.

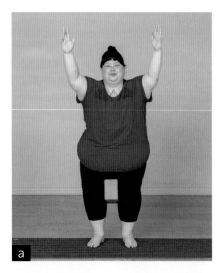

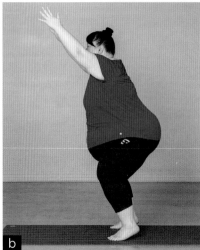

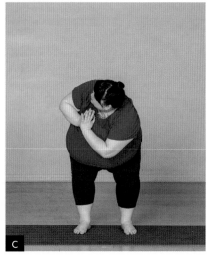

Figure 5.10 Accessible challenges for chair pose: *(a)* squeeze a block between the legs; *(b)* lift onto the balls of your feet and toes; *(c)* twist the torso to the right.

Tips for Plus-Sized Bodies

▦ Step your feet wider apart if your thighs need more space.

▦ Move your belly to each side during the twists to help you find your true range of motion.

Five-Pointed Star Pose (Utthita Tadasana)

Don't be fooled by how basic looking this pose is! Five-pointed star is a true power pose that can help you feel energy moving in your body in addition to all the other benefits. Like mountain pose, this posture is a great transition pose during your standing practice. I find that it's a nice time to check in with the breath and sensations in the body. Plus, it's a great starting position for tons of poses, which makes it a favorite of mine for both teaching and including in my personal practice.

Five-pointed star is a wonderful way to find expansiveness in your body. Since the limbs are unfurled and stretched long, you can ground yourself and extend out through your body to take up as much space as possible. I find this especially wonderful as someone who has spent her life being told to take up as little space as possible. I always keep that in mind when I practice this pose, reaching and stretching to make myself as big as I can!

Try five-pointed star and see what you can feel in your body. Look for sensations of lengthening, opening, and energizing through your whole body. This pose can also help with improving circulation and respiration because it lengthens and aligns the spine while opening the chest.

Alignment Checklist

- Begin in mountain pose. Step your feet wide apart and bring your arms out to each side.
- Rotating from the shoulders, turn your arms to face the front with palms forward.
- Press down evenly through each side of your feet: balls of the feet, heels, outer edges, and inner edges.
- Press firmly through your feet and pull up through your legs, but without locking your knees. Find a neutral position in your pelvis. Lengthen your torso and bring your shoulders back and down.
- Imagine a line dividing your body in two, from head to toe. Think of sending energy out from this midline through each limb. Reach out through the arms and legs and stretch as long as you can. Tuck your chin a tiny bit and lengthen the back of your neck (see figure 5.11).
- Hold here and keep muscles engaged while you extend out through the five points: arms, legs, and head. Stay for a few breaths or longer if you'd like.

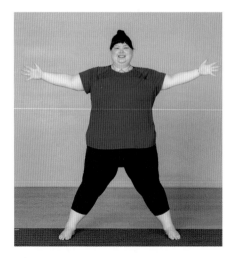

Figure 5.11 Five-pointed star pose.

Pose Options

■ Try bringing your palms together in front of your chest and extending out energetically through your elbows.

■ Sit on a chair, bringing your feet apart into a wide-leg position (see figure 5.12). All other instructions are the same as the standing version.

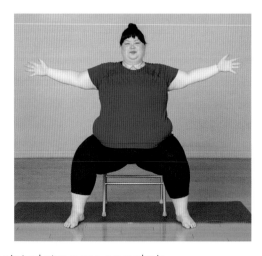

Figure 5.12 Five-pointed star pose on a chair.

Accessible Challenges

■ Add a balance element by raising up onto the balls of your feet or your toes.

■ Build extra strength by balancing blocks on your hands. Try turning your palms up and down to see how each way feels different.

■ Step the feet wider apart to work a little harder.

Triangle Pose (Trikonasana)

Triangle always feels like a Russian doll to me, where I think I know what it is and then realize there are more layers underneath. I find it a fascinating pose and come back to it often to play with variations and find new ways to experience it. The posture brings many elements together, though, at first, you may think it's merely a leg stretch. That's part of the appeal of the pose! There's always something new to focus on and feel.

Triangle is great at both stretching and strengthening your ankles, knees, and thighs. You can get deep stretches in your inner thighs, hips, back, and chest. You can build strength and stability in your feet, ankles, and legs. You can expand, open, and play with taking up space. You can even focus on finding balance in all areas of your body as you hold. Experiment with different intentions each time you practice triangle pose. Focus on body parts, your mental state and union with the body, breathing as you hold, and creating accessible challenges for yourself.

Alignment Checklist

- Begin in mountain pose and then step feet wider apart. Place a block, on its highest side, by your right foot. Turn your right leg 90 degrees out to the side, making sure to turn from your hip. Angle your left foot in slightly to the right. Your hips will be turned somewhat diagonally, but bring your shoulders and chest to face the front.

- Bend your right knee and then side-bend over to the right, bringing your right hand to the block. Twist your torso to face the front if it has moved out of alignment.

- Straighten your right leg so that both legs are straight and weight is evenly balanced between the two.

- Extend your left arm up toward the ceiling and either keep your head facing the front or turn your gaze to your left hand (see figure 5.13). Hold here for a few breaths.

- To come out of the pose, lower your left arm to your body and bring your gaze back to neutral. Bend your right knee and then press through your feet to bring your torso up to standing. Turn your toes forward and come to five-pointed star or return to mountain pose. Repeat triangle pose on the left side.

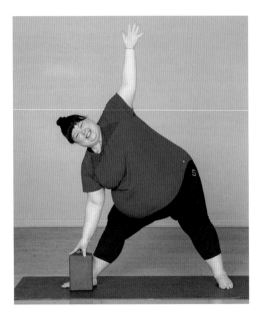

Figure 5.13 Triangle pose.

Pose Options

◼ Find support by standing in front of a wall (see figure 5.14). Instructions are the same, except that you make a stabilizing connection between the back of your torso and the wall.

◼ Instead of bringing your bottom hand to a block, try putting your hand on a chair seat.

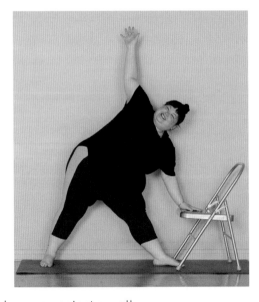

Figure 5.14 Triangle pose against a wall.

Accessible Challenges

■ Dial down the height of your block or practice triangle without support under your hand at all.

■ Step your feet wider apart to increase the challenge level.

Tips for Plus-Sized Bodies

Feel free to move your belly to make space when you twist your torso to the front.

Extended Side-Angle Pose (Utthita Parsvakonasana)

Extended side-angle builds off the alignment you find in triangle pose and brings in a deep opening for the side of the body. It's an excellent posture for the beginning of your practice to prepare the body for more intense poses afterward. With extended side-angle, you can find a lengthening in your sides, shoulders, chest, hips, and groin. It also strengthens and stretches your legs, knees, and ankles.

This is another pose, like triangle pose, where looks can be deceiving. Extended side-angle is not just a great transition pose (it is), but there are real benefits to be had. In addition to the strengthening and stretching it provides, the posture is also great for bringing a lot of accessible challenges to your practice. You can perform extended side-angle from a chair and find great challenges to fit your body's needs.

Alignment Checklist

■ Begin in mountain pose and then step the feet wider apart. Turn your right leg 90 degrees out to the side, making sure to turn from your hip. Angle your left foot slightly to the right. Your hips will be turned somewhat diagonally, but bring your shoulders and chest to face the front.

■ Bend your right knee, keeping your knee from going past your ankle, and then side-bend over to the right to bring your right forearm to your right thigh. Twist your torso to face the front if it has moved out of alignment. Your arm is resting on your thigh for support, but try not to dump all your weight onto it. Think of your thigh as something to push off from, not sink into.

■ Extend your left arm up and over to the right, stretching as long as you can from your fingers to your left foot (see figure 5.15). Keep your head in a neutral position, looking to the front. Hold here for a few breaths.

■ To come out of the pose, lower your left arm to your body and then press through your feet to bring your torso up to standing. Turn your toes forward and come to five-pointed star or return to mountain pose. Repeat extended side-angle pose on the left side.

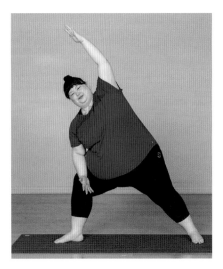

Figure 5.15 Extended side-angle pose.

Pose Options

■ Find support by standing in front of a wall. Instructions are the same, except that you make a stabilizing connection between the back of your torso and the wall.

■ Instead of bringing your bottom hand to your thigh, try putting your hand on a chair seat (see figure 5.16a).

■ Step your feet closer together.

■ Try the pose from seated on a chair (see figure 5.16b). Come to mountain pose on the chair and then step your feet wider apart. Extend your left leg out long to the side and then follow the instructions for extended side-angle.

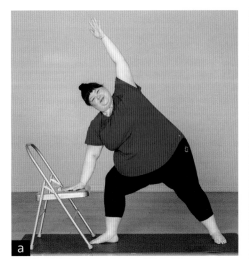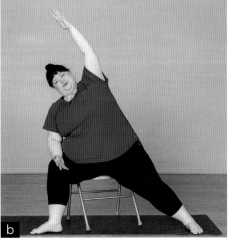

Figure 5.16 Extended side-angle pose on a chair: (a) hand on chair; (b) seated on chair.

Accessible Challenges

■ Lessen the amount of support you get from your forearm resting on your thigh. Or do not rest your forearm on your thigh at all and extend your bottom arm toward the floor.

■ Step your feet farther apart.

Tips for Plus-Sized Bodies

Feel free to move your belly to make space when you twist your torso to the front.

Warrior II Pose (Virabhadrasana II)

I think warrior II might be the world's most recognizable yoga pose. I have no evidence other than seeing it used everywhere to sell things from yogurt to vacations. What is the appeal of the pose? Why does it feel so yoga-y to practice it? My guess is that it's the expansion of the limbs, the strength you can see, the grounding element, and the graceful, focused movement. Try it out and see if you can nail down why it's such a popular pose.

The posture certainly brings a lot of benefits to the table! Practicing warrior II can strengthen and stretch your arms, shoulders, chest, hips, thighs, ankles, and feet. You can engage your muscles and hold, strengthening and improving your stamina. Or you can find some gentle movement and bring fluidity and softness to your practice. Warrior II can be practiced from standing and from sitting on a chair. You can add elements to level up and find accessible challenges that fit any need you might have.

Alignment Checklist

■ Begin in mountain pose and then step feet wider apart. Turn your right leg 90 degrees out to the side, making sure to turn from your hip. Angle your left foot in slightly to the right. Your hips will be turned somewhat diagonally, but bring your shoulders and chest to face the front.

■ Bend your right knee, keeping your knee from going past your ankle. If you'd like to bend the knee more, you can step your left foot farther away and maintain alignment.

■ Bring your arms up and out to each side, with palms facing down. Keep your weight evenly distributed and your torso straight up. If your left shoulder has moved forward, press it back to keep a straight line from your right fingertips to your chest to the left fingertips. Turn your head to the right and look out over your fingers (see figure 5.17).

■ Hold here for a few breaths and then come out by straightening your right leg, turning your toes forward, and coming to five-pointed star or returning to mountain pose. Repeat warrior II on the left side.

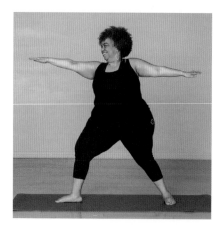

Figure 5.17 Warrior II pose.

Pose Options

▥ Try the pose from seated on a chair (see figure 5.18). Come to mountain pose on the chair and then step your feet wider apart. Extend your left leg out long to the side and then follow the instructions for warrior II.

▥ Step your feet closer together.

▥ Try positioning your arms differently to relieve shoulder strain or experience the pose in a new way. Bring palms together at your chest and extend energetically through your elbows.

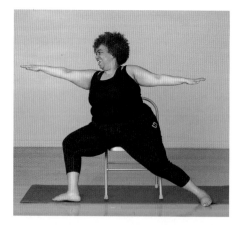

Figure 5.18 Warrior II pose on a chair.

Accessible Challenges

▥ Hold the pose and send energy out through your front shin and back leg. Press each direction and notice how it feels in your body.

▥ Step your feet farther apart to hold more weight and work harder.

Deep-Squat Pose (Malasana)

I once read somewhere that we should be practicing this squat every day for five minutes, and, for some reason, that has stuck with me for years. I like to sprinkle this pose in while I'm doing chores around the house, and I've found it fits right in when I'm taking clothes out of the dryer, watering my plants outside, dusting low shelves and spaces, and playing with my cats. I don't know if everyone needs to practice this every day, but it's working for me!

Deep-squat can help you find great flexibility in your ankles, inner thighs, and back. It's gently strengthening for your legs and core and a great hip-opening posture. However, please be gentle with yourself. This pose is not for those folks with compromised hips, knees, or ankles. If you try this and find discomfort or pain in those or any other areas, stop immediately.

Alignment Checklist

- Begin in mountain pose. Turn your feet out slightly and squat down, bringing your tailbone down toward the ground (see figure 5.19).
- Adjust your stance if needed. You can bring the feet farther apart or closer together, depending on what feels better for your body.
- Keep your torso lifted and tall, which should help to press your tailbone down toward the floor.
- Try to press your heels down to the floor, but don't force them. Your arms can rest on your thighs, palms can come together at your chest, or you can raise your arms overhead with palms facing each other.
- Hold for a few breaths or longer if that feels safe. To come out of the pose, inhale and straighten the knees, coming back up to mountain pose.

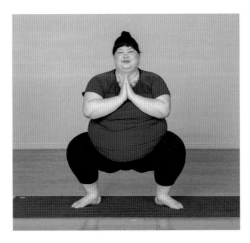

Figure 5.19 Deep-squat pose.

Pose Options

■ If your heels don't reach the floor, place a rolled blanket underneath them for support (see figure 5.20a).

■ A stack of blocks or a firm bolster underneath your sit bones will give great support and allow you to hold the pose longer (see figure 5.20b).

■ Practice this pose while seated on a chair (see figure 5.20c) to get the benefits without the struggle. Sit on the front edge of your chair and place your feet on top of a stack of blocks, bolsters, pillows, folded blankets, or whatever else you have on hand. You can experiment to find the height of support that works for you. Keep your torso tall and bring your hands to the chair back or seat if you need extra stability.

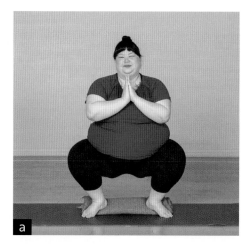

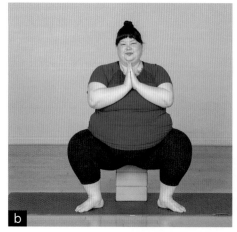
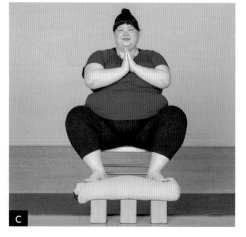

Figure 5.20 Deep-squat pose options: (a) rolled blanket under the heels; (b) stack of blocks under the sit bones; (c) deep-squat on a chair.

Accessible Challenges

- Work your heels all the way down to the floor.
- Sink your tailbone lower and lift your torso higher.
- Bring your arms overhead or wrap them around your legs from the outside and reach for each ankle from the inside.

Tips for Plus-Sized Bodies

Feel free to move your belly to the center to make space for your thighs.

Warrior III Pose (Virabhadrasana III)

Let me start by reminding you that whatever version of the pose you do is exactly right. Why the disclaimer? Warrior III is an intimidating pose even to those of us with years of practice behind us. It's a balance pose that both requires and builds strength. Often, the only version you see represented is the full-on, most difficult form. If that's something you want to work toward, great! However, I want you to know that there are many ways to practice warrior III. I'm excited to show you some of them!

The benefits of warrior III are many, including building strength, stability, and balance. This is a full-body pose, and you might feel it the next day. Be gentle and patient with yourself. It may take some time and practice to balance for longer than a couple of breaths. You'll probably fall out of the pose a bunch of times. Take it slowly and move at your own pace. It's not a competition!

Alignment Checklist

▥ Begin in mountain pose. Shift your weight into your right leg, bending your left knee and resting only the toes of your left foot on the floor. Find your balance here before you move to the next step.

▥ Slide your left foot back until the leg is straight but your toes are still on the ground. Keep your right knee soft, taking care to not lock the knee.

▥ Raise your arms overhead with palms facing each other. Move your arms forward until they make a straight line from your fingers to your left foot. Think of your body as a seesaw.

▥ Engage the muscles in your core, legs, and arms. Begin to slowly lift your left leg off the floor any amount (see figure 5.21a). Be sure to mirror the movement with your torso. As your leg lifts, your torso should come forward (see figure 5.21b). Keep the straight line of your body at all times. Lift your leg only as much as feels like a personal challenge for you. A low leg is just as valid as a higher leg in this pose. They're both balance poses.

▥ Keep your hips facing forward the whole time. As you lift your leg, the hips should remain forward. It is often helpful to think of keeping your toes and knee pointed forward and down. You don't want your toes or knee to face the side.

▥ Hold here as long as you like. To come out of the pose, seesaw your leg down and torso up. Come back into mountain pose. Repeat on the left side.

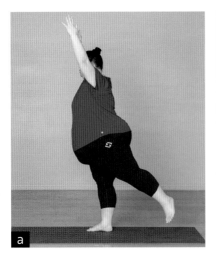 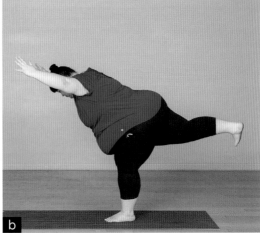

Figure 5.21 Warrior III pose options: *(a)* low-leg option; *(b)* higher-leg option.

Pose Options

■ For more support, follow the instructions for warrior III but bring your hands to a chair seat or chair back (see figure 5.22). You can keep both arms on the support or take turns lifting and reaching forward with one arm at a time.

■ Try bringing the raised foot to rest on a wall or chair seat. You can add this support alone or combine it with bringing the hands to a chair.

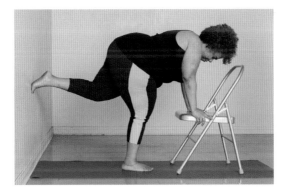

Figure 5.22 Warrior III pose on a chair.

Accessible Challenges

Play with lifting your leg higher or using less support.

Tips for Plus-Sized Bodies

Remember you can always step your feet wider to make space for your thighs. If your thighs are pressed against each other, it can put you off balance from the start.

High-Lunge Pose (Alanasana)

This is a great posture that works at the beginning or end of your practice. Since it prepares the body for more intense poses, it's often taught toward the start of a standing sequence. That doesn't mean you have to stick to that! Try putting this pose into your sequences wherever you need a good leg stretching or strengthening. Add in a backbend, and you've got a full-body pose that is easy to tailor to your specific needs.

High-lunge can stretch and strengthen your back, shoulders, and leg muscles. It opens your hips and chest and is great at stretching your groin and increasing mobility in your hip flexors. Add in the practice with balancing, and you've got the whole package!

Alignment Checklist

■ Begin in mountain pose. Step your left foot forward and then adjust your stride as needed by stepping your right foot backward, with the ball of the foot on the floor. Step back far enough so that your left knee can bend as deeply as you want.

■ Raise your arms overhead with palms facing each other and hinge your torso forward slightly so that your body makes a straight line from your fingers to your right heel (see figure 5.23).

■ Keep your hips and toes facing forward. Stretch your right heel down toward the floor.

■ Hold for a few breaths and come out of the pose by stepping your back foot forward and resuming mountain pose. Repeat on the other side.

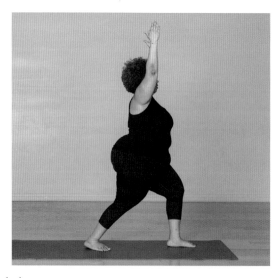

Figure 5.23   High-lunge pose.

Pose Options

▥ Step your feet closer together to shorten your stride or wider apart to find more stability.

▥ Place a block between your front knee and a wall to practice extending energetically forward and find some support (see figure 5.24a).

▥ Keep your torso more upright instead of leaning forward.

▥ Practice the pose with a chair seat under your front thigh for support. If needed, place a block under the front foot to raise the floor up and provide stability.

▥ Find support for the upper body and increased stability by bringing your hands to a chair seat (see figure 5.24b).

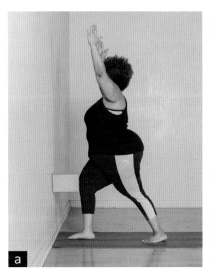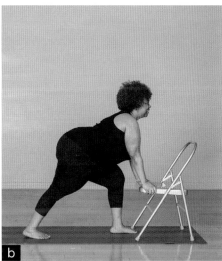

Figure 5.24   High-lunge pose options: *(a)* with a block; *(b)* with a chair.

Accessible Challenges

▥ Add a backbend as you're holding the pose.

▥ Step your feet farther apart to lengthen your stride.

CONCLUSION

Well look at you! You've made it through the standing poses and are well on your way to an awesome yoga practice. How are you feeling? I wouldn't be surprised if you felt accomplished, proud, and maybe even a little excited about what you've learned and what is yet to come. These standing poses are such great tools to stash in your yoga asana toolbox! You can use these by themselves or in combination with the seated and kneeling poses from the previous chapter and with the reclined postures that are coming up next.

What did you think of these standing poses? Were there any that you have lingering questions about or want to research to find out more about them? Give yourself permission to want to know more! The learning doesn't stop with this book; this is just the beginning of your lifelong study of yoga. Take a moment to think about the postures from this chapter. Which did you like best, worst, feel confused about, or look forward to experimenting with? Were you already familiar with any of them? This is the perfect time to check in with yourself about how you're feeling now that you've gotten this far into the book. Maybe now would be a good time to stop and journal about how you're feeling or share with a friend. I encourage you to reflect on and express the thoughts and feelings that are coming up as you work through the book. There's so much information coming at you and lots of new ideas to process and absorb. It's natural to need a little space to sort through what you're feeling and thinking. Take a break! Press pause and come back later if that feels right. Self-care is an important part of your yoga practice!

I'm very excited to tell you that coming up in the next chapter are some of my favorites: reclined poses! I think sometimes people think that reclined poses are all super easy, relaxation-focused postures, but that's not true at all. I mean, yes, some of them are restorative poses, and they're glorious! However, not all of them are about relaxing, and I think it's really cool to have the different types of poses accessible from a reclined position. In the next chapter, you'll find an assortment of my favorite reclined poses that require some more active work in the body. There are backbends, core strengtheners, and some great stretches coming your way. If you're disappointed and were hoping for the restorative poses, skip to chapter 7!

CHAPTER 6

RECLINED POSES

There are many reasons why we should include reclined postures in our practices. I find them incredibly helpful for adding gentle backbends, strengthening, and stretching into my sequences. As both a practitioner and teacher of yoga, I love the impact these poses can have on the body without much of the strain or struggle that can come with standing versions. There are both upward- and downward-facing poses in this chapter. Together, they give a holistic sampling of the many benefits you can find with floor poses.

Reclined poses are excellent to practice when you want to work on flexibility. I've included some accessible backbends here to help you find more ease and movement in your back and hips. They all pair well and can be practiced as a sequence if you want! The poses included are also helpful in gaining strength in gentle ways, with you in control of the depth and intensity of the movements. I love all the poses in this chapter because they bring the support that allows you to focus on your alignment in a mindful way.

This chapter is organized a bit differently from the others, with four single-pose explanations and then a series of poses explained together. The series you'll find within is explained to you in exactly the way I practice and teach these poses. Of course, you can play with these poses individually. I also encourage you to try them together to see how they build on each other and provide a great series to bring your practice to an end.

Each pose in the chapter has its own section with a detailed explanation of all aspects of the pose, including the following:

- The benefits the pose can bring to your body and mind
- An alignment checklist, step-by-step instructions for how to get into the pose, and what sensations to look for in your body to know that you have the correct alignment
- Pose options to tailor the pose to work for your body as it is in that moment
- Ways to create accessible challenges for yourself, if you want to
- Any plus-size-specific tips that apply to the pose

Sphinx Pose (Salamba Bhujangasana)

Sphinx pose is a gentle backbend that can help you open and stretch your chest, shoulders, and back. Performed on the forearms, it's particularly helpful for folks who have wrist pain, stiffness, or injury that makes putting pressure on the wrists painful or impossible. Your body gets support from your forearms to help lift the torso into a small backbend. Remember to use the rest of your body to help support! The arms shouldn't be doing all the work.

While the pose is a gentle backbend, it's not only for newer practitioners. Sphinx pose is also good for practicing proper alignment and strength building for those with more experience. Sphinx and the following pose, cobra (page 127), are often performed together as a progression. I love them together and encourage you to try them in this way and notice how it feels to practice these in a sequence. You can perform them with more support for a gentle backbend or less support for an accessible challenge!

Alignment Checklist

■ Lie on your belly with your forearms on the floor, palms down, in front of you. Align your elbows underneath your shoulders. Extend your legs out long, close together, with the tops of your feet on the floor. Send energy down your legs and out through your toes to keep your legs engaged.

■ Inhale and lift your forehead, chin, and chest, coming into a small backbend (see figure 6.1). Press gently through your whole forearms, including all the way to your fingertips. Try not to hold all your weight in your elbows. Think of your arms, shoulders, and chest as a frame that holds the body. Engage your whole upper body to help hold the weight of your torso.

■ Bring your gaze diagonally to the floor in front of you so that the back of your neck is long.

■ Engage the muscles of your core to help hold you in this lifted position. Then, moving down the body, gently engage your muscles to assist in holding your lifted torso. You want to engage, not clench, your muscles. Try pressing the tops of your feet down onto the floor.

■ Hold here for a few breaths or as long as it feels like a personal challenge for you. To come out of the pose, exhale and lower your chest, chin, and then forehead down to the mat or a folded blanket. Repeat as many times as you like. You can follow this with cobra for a backbend progression if you want.

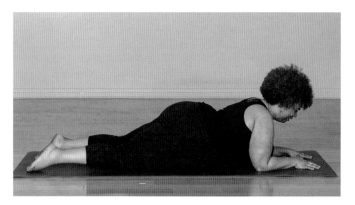

Figure 6.1 Sphinx pose.

Pose Options

▓ Get some support for lifting your torso by placing a folded blanket underneath your ribs.

▓ Try practicing sphinx pose against a wall from a standing position (see figure 6.2). Come to mountain pose in front of a wall. Follow the instructions for sphinx pose, keeping your feet flat on the ground and pressing away from the wall to find your gentle backbend.

▓ If the backbend feels too intense, you can slide your forearms forward, away from your chest, to lessen the arch in your back.

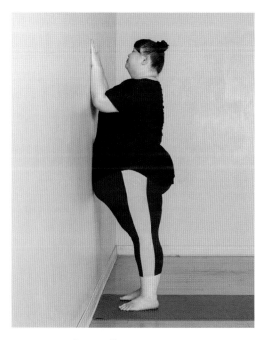

Figure 6.2 Sphinx pose on the wall.

Accessible Challenges

Experiment by using less support from your arms, working your way up to no support at all. Come into alignment and then lift your forearms off the floor any distance. Use the rest of your body to support the lift in your torso and hold as long as it feels like a challenge for you.

Tips for Plus-Sized Bodies

■ If you feel your belly and thighs compressing in an uncomfortable way, try this option. Tuck your toes under and lift your knees and thighs up away from the floor. Press your heels away toward the wall behind you so that your legs move down. Lower your thighs and knees back to the floor and untuck your toes. This can help to clear the feeling of congestion that occurs when your belly and thighs meet at your hips when the body is in a prone position.

■ If your breasts are uncomfortable or keep you from lying flat on your belly, place a folded blanket underneath your ribs and a block underneath your forehead.

Cobra (Bhujangasana)

Cobra is another great backbend that can be performed on the floor or a wall, making it a wonderfully accessible posture for all yogis. It can help you stretch your chest while also strengthening your spine and shoulders. I find that it helps me feel both calm and more energized! Like sphinx pose, cobra activates the whole body and can be practiced as a gentle backbend or a strengthening pose depending on what you need.

Alignment Checklist

■ Lie on your belly with your hands on the floor, palms down, underneath your shoulders. Hug your elbows into your sides. Extend your legs out long, close together, with the tops of your feet on the floor. Send energy down your legs and out through your toes to keep your legs engaged.

■ Inhale and lift your forehead, chin, and chest, coming into a backbend. Press very gently through your hands, letting the backbend come naturally without being forced (see figure 6.3). Lift your torso into a backbend but keep the front of your hips on the floor. If pressing up until the arms straighten causes your hips to lift off the floor, bend your elbows a little. Think of your arms, shoulders, and chest as a frame that holds the body. Engage your whole upper body to help hold the weight of your torso.

■ Bring your gaze diagonally to the floor in front of you so that the back of your neck is long. If you feel comfortable, you can experiment with lifting your gaze toward the ceiling, but be careful not to collapse the back of the neck. Keep your shoulders away from your ears.

■ Engage the muscles of your core to help hold you in this lifted position. Then, moving down the body, gently engage your muscles to assist in holding your lifted torso. You want to engage, not clench, your muscles. Try pressing the tops of your feet down onto the floor.

■ Hold for a few breaths or as long as feels like a personal challenge for you. To come out of the pose, exhale and lower your chest, chin, and then forehead down to the mat or a folded blanket. Repeat as many times as you like.

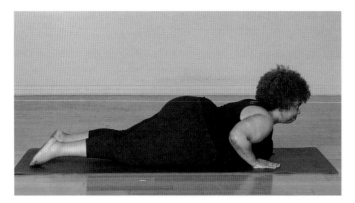

Figure 6.3   Cobra pose.

Pose Options

■ Get some support when lifting your torso by placing a folded blanket underneath your ribs.

■ Try practicing cobra pose against a wall from a standing position (see figure 6.4). Come to mountain pose in front of a wall. Follow the instructions for cobra, keeping your feet flat on the ground and pressing away from the wall to find your gentle backbend.

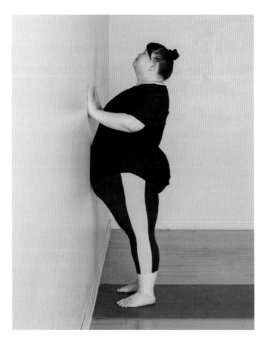

Figure 6.4   Cobra pose against a wall.

Accessible Challenges

Experiment by using less support from your arms, working your way up to no support at all. Come into alignment and then lift your hands off the floor any distance. Use the rest of your body to support the lift in your torso and hold as long as it feels like a challenge for you.

Tips for Plus-Sized Bodies

- If you feel your belly and thighs compressing in an uncomfortable way, try this option. Tuck your toes under and lift your knees and thighs up away from the floor. Press your heels away toward the wall behind you so that your legs move down. Lower your thighs and knees back to the floor and untuck your toes. This can help to clear the feeling of congestion that occurs when your belly and thighs meet at your hips when the body is in a prone position.

- If your breasts are uncomfortable or keep you from lying flat on your belly, place a folded blanket underneath your ribs and a block underneath your forehead.

Locust Pose (Salabhasana)

Locust pose is both another belly-down backbend and also a great option to build strength in your whole body. While it's tempting to focus only on the flexibility to be gained, I want to make sure you know how helpful this pose can be in gaining strength from an accessible floor position. Locust is a winner in my book because of the support from underneath and the many options available to customize it. Depending on how you move your legs and upper body, you can find the level of challenge and support that honors your body's needs.

Like sphinx and cobra poses, locust is a great preparatory pose for deeper backbends and more intense movement later in your practice. Try including it in the beginning of your sequence to warm the body and also at the end to counter any poses that came before. Locust pose increases flexibility and strengthens both the front and back sides of the body. It's truly an impactful pose that fits into any yogi's practice. Experiment with moving in and out of the pose with your breath, inhaling as you come up and exhaling as you come down. Or hold in the lifted position for extra strengthening. There are lots of adjustments and options for locust pose, which helps to keep your practice fun and fresh!

Alignment Checklist

■ Lie on your belly with your forehead resting on your mat or a folded blanket and your arms down by your sides. Make sure the tops of your feet are on the floor and not tucked under.

■ Inhale, lifting your right leg straight up toward the ceiling. Keep your leg straight, with pointed toes, and extend it long behind you. Don't worry about how high you're lifting the leg, just focus on keeping your hips, knee, and top of your foot facing the mat. Exhale and bring the leg gently back down to the floor. Repeat on the left side. Try making the same movement, but with both legs at one time (see figure 6.5a). Focus on lifting and keeping the legs straight and toes pointed and reaching away.

■ Now, let your legs rest and bring your attention to your upper body. Inhale, lifting your forehead, chin, chest, and arms off the floor (see figure 6.5b). Keep your gaze straight ahead so you don't collapse through the back of your neck. Reach back with your arms and lift your chest up to find a backbend. Exhale back to the floor and bring your arms, chest, chin, and then forehead to rest on the mat.

■ Try putting it all together! Inhale, lifting torso, arms, and legs up as high as it feels comfortable (see figure 6.5c). Exhale down or hold for a few breaths. Repeat as many times as you like.

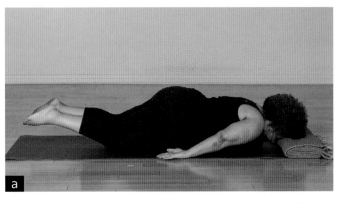

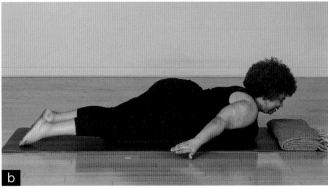

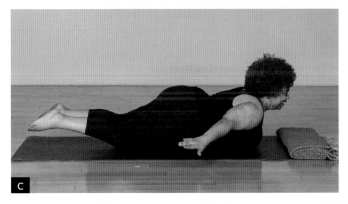

Figure 6.5 Locust pose: *(a)* lift both legs; *(b)* lift upper body; *(c)* lift legs and upper body.

Pose Options

▥ Get some support when lifting your torso or legs by placing a folded blanket underneath your ribs or thighs.

▥ If lifting both legs isn't working for you, isolate each leg one at a time. Or if lifting both your upper and lower body together isn't working, isolate each section one at a time.

Accessible Challenges

- Level up by holding any combination of your upper and lower body for longer lengths of time.
- Stretch your arms out long in front of you and hold them there while you lift your torso.

Tips for Plus-Sized Bodies

- If you feel your belly and thighs compressing in an uncomfortable way, try this option. Tuck your toes under and lift your knees and thighs up away from the floor. Press your heels away toward the wall behind you so that your legs move down. Lower your thighs and knees back to the floor and untuck your toes. This can help to clear the feeling of congestion that occurs when your belly and thighs meet at your hips when the body is in a prone position.
- If your breasts are uncomfortable or keep you from lying flat on your belly, place a folded blanket underneath your ribs and a block underneath your forehead.

Bridge Pose (Setu Bandha Sarvangasana)

Bridge pose was a game changer for me, and I hope it can enrich your practice as well. The posture is good for energizing the body and bringing strength and flexibility to your back, hips, legs, ankles, and feet. However, it can also be a wonderfully rejuvenating pose that fits into a calming restorative practice. I'll dig into bridge as a restorative pose in the next chapter, but, for now, let's focus on the other great characteristics it has. The crucial help I found with bridge pose was in finding a way to prepare my body to lie flat on the floor. Before I added the posture to my practice regularly, I found being on my back on the floor to be uncomfortable and sometimes even impossible. By practicing both the active and restorative versions of the pose, I was able to stretch my spine and front body in a way that changed lying supine for me forever!

Bridge pose stretches the neck, chest, spine, hips, thighs, and ankles. It brings your heart higher than your head, which helps to make you feel calm and can bring some relief from headaches. I find it to be an energizing pose that feels great after a long day of sitting at the computer.

Alignment Checklist

- Lie on your back with your knees bent and the soles of your feet on the floor. Step your feet and knees hip-distance apart. Place your arms by your sides with palms facing down.
- Inhaling, press through your arms and feet and lift your hips off the floor (see figure 6.6). Don't worry about how high you lift your hips. You can always play with finding more height later.
- Be sure to press through your whole foot, including the toes and inner edges of your feet. Also press though your whole arms, including through your fingers.
- Exhale, gently lowering your hips back to the floor. Move up and down a few times, matching your movements to your breath.
- Inhale, bringing hips up, and hold for a few breaths. As you hold, keep breathing. You may like to step your feet in closer toward your torso. Often, this can help to make space for lifting the hips higher. Notice how the weight you're holding shifts higher up toward your shoulders as you lift your hips higher.
- You can keep your arms where they are or choose to move them. Try bringing the hands underneath your hips and clasping the palms together, fingers intertwined. Or roll your arms out to tuck your shoulders underneath your body and bring the shoulder blades closer together. Then, ground your elbows into the floor and bring the palms of your hands to your hips to support them as you hold.
- When you're ready, exhale and bring your hips down to the floor. Rock your knees side to side to clear tension from your hips and lower back. Repeat as many times as you like.

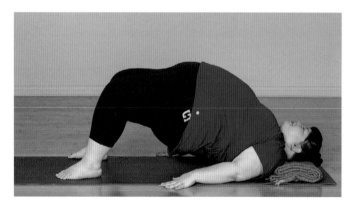

Figure 6.6 Bridge pose.

Pose Options

■ Try a version where the hips stay connected to the ground. The instructions for setup are the same. Instead of pressing through the feet and arms and lifting your hips completely off the floor, lift and keep a connection. This way you get some support from the floor while still engaging your whole body.

■ Follow the same setup instructions. Instead of lifting your hips, tilt your pelvis forward and backward (see figure 6.7), moving with your breath. Inhale, tilting the base of your pelvis up and forward and then exhale and switch directions to tilt it down and backward.

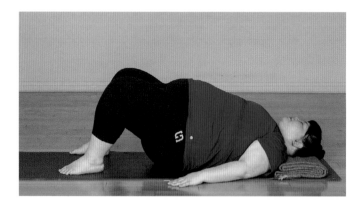

Figure 6.7 Bridge pose with pelvis tilt.

Accessible Challenges

As you hold your lifted hips in bridge pose, lift a leg off the floor. You can keep it low or bring the foot up toward the ceiling. Switch legs.

Wind-Reliever Series (Pavanamuktasana Series)

This series is one of my favorite sequences to teach and practice myself! I learned a version of this from Abby Lentz from HeavyWeight Yoga and have put my own spin on it over the years. It's now the way we prepare for savasana, deep-relaxation pose, in all of my classes. I love how each person who tries it finds something helpful for herself. I encourage you to try these poses alone and as a series. There is something wonderful about how they all flow together and help to stretch the body to release tension and bring relief from tight muscles. The following poses make up the wind-reliever series: knees-to-chest, reclining hand-to-big-toe, supine twist, reclining straddle, happy baby, and floating bound-angle. It sounds like a lot, but, once you learn them all, you'll see how they work and make sense together!

As the name suggests, the wind-reliever series is helpful in releasing tension from your muscles and unwanted gas from your digestive system. It's also helpful in relieving indigestion, bloating, and pain associated with menstrual cramps and sciatica. I teach this series at the end of every class as a way to transition to stillness. The series does a nice job wringing excess energy and tension from the body in order to help you find stillness and rest in our final deep-relaxation pose.

Alignment Checklist

▪ Knees-to-chest pose (pavanamuktasana): See figure 6.8a. Lie on your back with your feet on the floor and knees pointed toward the ceiling. Lift your legs up and wrap a strap around the balls of your feet, holding one end of the strap in each hand. Pull on the strap, bringing your knees as far into your chest as possible. Hold here and lift your forehead toward your knees for a few breaths. As you hold, rock forward and backward or side to side if it feels good to do so. When ready, bring your left foot out of the strap and put it back on the floor.

▪ Reclining hand-to-big-toe pose (supta padangusthasana): See figures 6.8b and 6.8c. Keep your right foot in the strap and lift it toward the ceiling. Straighten your leg as much as necessary to feel a stretch up the back of the leg. Keep the right foot flexed to find the most stretch possible. Your left leg can be bent or straight, whichever is more comfortable for you. Hold here for a few breaths and then move both ends of the strap to your right hand. Place your left arm out to the side for support and then lower your right leg out to the side. Use the strap to hold the weight of your leg.

Keep your left hip firmly down on the floor to get the best stretch for your inner thighs. Hold here for a few breaths and then inhale and lift your right leg toward the ceiling again.

▥ Supine twist pose (supta matsyendrasana): See figure 6.8d. Grab both ends of the strap with your left hand and place your right arm out to the side, palm down, for support. Using your strap, guide your right leg across your body and over to the left. Keep your right shoulder down to the floor but allow your right hip to come up. Find the twist in your spine and the stretch in your outer hip and thigh. Hold here for a few breaths and then inhale and lift your right leg toward the ceiling again.

▥ Bring your left leg up into the strap and then place your right foot down on the floor. Repeat everything on the left side.

▥ Reclining straddle pose (supta upavistha konasana): See figure 6.8e. Bring your right foot back into the strap to join the left one and hold one end of the strap in each hand. Now that both feet are in the strap, slide them apart toward each end of your strap, opening your legs out into the widest V you can make. Straighten your legs and pull on each end of the strap to bring your feet toward your head. This should be a deep stretch for your inner thighs. Try rocking side to side as you hold the stretch for a few breaths.

▥ Happy baby pose (ananda balasana): See figure 6.8f. Slide your feet a little closer together within the strap. Bend your knees and pull the strap straight down with each hand until your knees come closer to your chest. Keep your feet flexed with the soles of your feet facing the ceiling. Hold here for a few breaths without moving or add a gentle rocking motion from side to side or forward and backward.

▥ Floating bound-angle pose (supta baddha konasana): See figure 6.8g. Straighten the legs and open your legs out from the hips so that your knees point out. Bring the soles of your feet together and loop your strap around the outside edges of your feet and on top of your ankles so that you can hold each end and support the weight of your legs. Gently pull the strap toward you and down as far as feels good to you. Hold here for a few breaths and then release the strap and bring your feet down to the floor. Rock your knees side to side to clear any tension from your hips and lower back.

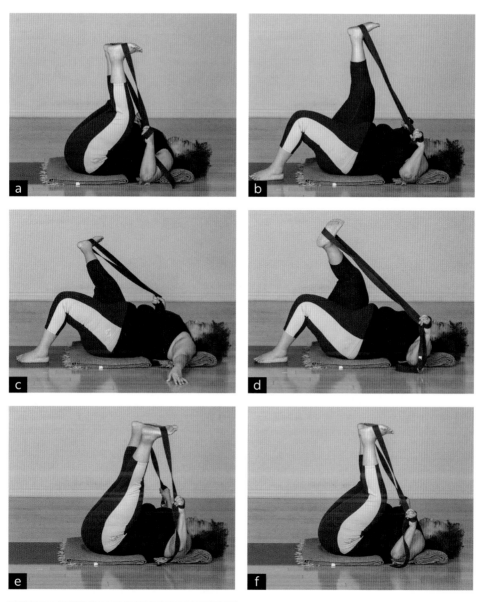

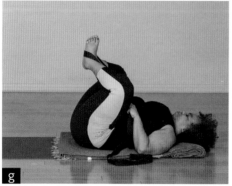

Figure 6.8 Wind-reliever series: (a) knees-to-chest pose; (b) reclining hand-to-big-toe pose, foot toward ceiling; (c) reclining hand-to-big-toe pose, foot to side; (d) supine twist pose; (e) reclining straddle pose; (f) happy baby pose; (g) floating bound-angle pose.

> ### *Tips for Plus-Sized Bodies*
>
> ■ In knees-to-chest, happy baby, and floating bound-angle, widen your feet and knees to the sides of your belly and pull down on the strap to get your knees closer to your chest if you find your knees meet your belly and can't move forward any more.
>
> ■ In reclining hand-to-big-toe, you can open your knee out to the side to act as a counterweight to the extended leg. Sometimes the weight of the extended leg, even with the strap's support, pulls down and makes the opposite hip leave the ground. Opening the other knee out to the side, like one-half of bound-angle pose, can balance the weight distribution and make it easier to stay in alignment.
>
> ■ In supine twist, use your free hand to sweep your belly up and away if the top thigh is meeting the belly and isn't able to find its full range of motion.

CONCLUSION

Whoa, another chapter down and more poses in your toolbox! I hope these reclined poses didn't disappoint. I love how they bring a different set of sensations and challenges to the mat than seated and standing poses. There's something about being reclined on your back or your belly to change how you experience stretches and strengthening postures. What did you think? Have you tried any of these before? I hope you can give yourself all the credit for learning so many new things as you move through the book. This is a lot of information and can feel overwhelming sometimes, especially if you're totally new to the world of yoga.

Which postures in this chapter were your favorites? Did any stick out as extra interesting or appealing? Take a little time to sort through your thoughts and get clear on how you're feeling right now. Remember that you can always book-mark your spot and come back later when you feel ready to move on or revisit the chapter. I know I say this all the time, but it can be overwhelming to learn so many new things at one time! Be patient with yourself and proud of all the awesome new information you've learned.

One of the cool things about adding more postures to your toolbox is that it means your practice can be even more diverse and interesting. More poses equals more interesting! These reclined poses bring a different element to your practice than the previous chapters' poses, and the learning doesn't stop here. Let's recap! You've learned about centering and breath work, seated and kneeling poses, standing postures, and reclined poses. What's missing here?

I hope you guessed restorative poses because that's what's coming up in the next chapter! If this is what you've been waiting for, then I am so excited for you! Let's dive into some great poses to bring relaxing, calm, and peaceful energy into your life. Be sure to do anything you need to prepare your body and your mind to keep going. Take a break, drink some water, go for a walk, and when you're ready, let's get relaxed!

RESTORATIVE POSES

The poses in this chapter are a different type than the others you've seen in the book so far. Restorative poses are all about embracing slowness and giving your body permission to gently open and release. These postures call for the support of blocks, blankets, bolsters or firm pillows, straps, a wall, a chair, and anything else that might support your body. Practicing restorative poses is different from the more active postures you might be used to. Think of practicing these poses as a mental and physical break from the rest of your life. A restorative practice may include only a few poses held for more time. In fact, I often add a little restorative practice to my workday with only one pose that I hold for 10 to 15 minutes. These are great postures to fit into your day to bring relief from tight muscles, poor posture, and the stresses of your life. The best part is that you can completely customize them to fit your life and needs! Your practice can adapt to fit any circumstance. I like to practice a restorative pose after I get off a plane and make it to my hotel room. It's a wonderful way to transition from traveling and help reduce my stress and any swelling of my feet and ankles. I even use restorative practices during road trips and while staying at a friend's house. This practice is yours to use any time you need it.

The poses in this chapter can be held for as long as feels good to you. In the beginning, it might be best to aim for 5 to 10 minutes and see how you feel. Some folks find restorative yoga poses to be relaxing and rejuvenating, and they are happy to hold them for upwards of 20 minutes. However, not everyone finds it easy to relax into these poses. You may find that you struggle to release your control and hold on your mind and body. Don't worry if that happens! The struggle is very common, but you will eventually find greater ease and release in restorative poses.

Some of these postures are supported versions of reclined or seated poses we've covered already. The added support of blocks, bolsters, blankets, and straps helps to eliminate unnecessary straining and struggling and allow you to sink into the stretch with ease. For example, supported bridge pose is adapted from the active version by adding support under the hips to hold you in position. That way you can relax into the posture and get the benefits without the struggle of holding yourself up. Another supported version we'll be digging into is supported fish, a pose we haven't covered anywhere else in this book. Honestly, I never teach any other version of fish pose. I don't see a need to do so when all the benefits can be had, and in a safer way, through the supported version.

It can be nice to dim the lights, play soothing music, and wear cozy clothing for your restorative practice. You might want to have an extra blanket on hand to cover your body during the long holds. It's challenging to relax when you're chilly. Also, an eye pillow is a very nice touch for restorative poses. The gentle weight of an eye pillow stimulates the vagus nerve and helps to calm you and reduce stress in the body. Despite the gentle and soothing nature of a restorative practice, don't be surprised if you find that you feel sore or can notice the effects of the poses the next day. These postures are restoring, but they're also very effective passive stretches!

Each pose in the chapter has its own section with a detailed explanation of all aspects of the pose, including the following:

- The benefits the pose can bring to your body and mind
- An alignment checklist, step-by-step instructions for how to get into the pose, and what sensations to look for in your body to know that you have the correct alignment
- Pose options to tailor the pose to work for your body as it is in that moment
- Ways to create accessible challenges for yourself, if you want to
- Any plus-size-specific tips that apply to the pose

Supported Bridge Pose (Salamba Setu Bandha Sarvangasana)

I discussed my experiences with the active version of bridge pose in chapter 6, and I'm excited to tell you about the supported restorative option. As I mentioned before, bridge pose was a game changer for me. Practicing it has helped my body find ease and comfort while lying on my back. Not only that, but the posture has given me freedom and opened up possibilities to stretch, strengthen, and move more in a supine position. Like many folks, I find holding my legs in the air while on my back to be a challenge. I can do it, but it takes a lot of core strength, and I lose any restorative benefit I was searching for. This pose gives the body support and changes the angles of your hips to make holding your legs up less demanding.

I'm hoping that supported bridge pose can be the comforting accessible posture for you that it has been for me. The pose can be calming, restoring, grounding, and centering. Depending on your leg position, you can get a front-body stretch that combats the tightness that comes with sitting for a long time. I find this particularly helpful when I've been working at the computer all day or driving a lot. You can lift the legs in the air to find movement or stillness that can ease tired and swollen legs. There are many different leg and arm positions that can help to ease a range of discomforts and body woes. Additionally, the pose can be combined with breathing and meditation techniques to help ease and calm your mind.

Alignment Checklist

- Lie on your back next to your bolster with your knees bent and the soles of your feet on the floor. Step your feet and knees hip-distance apart. Place your arms by your sides with palms down.
- Inhale, pressing through your arms and feet as you lift your hips off the floor. Hold your hips up and slide your bolster underneath you.
- Exhale, gently lowering your hips to the bolster (see figure 7.1). Make any necessary adjustments to your position. Position the top edge of the bolster in the dip of your lower back for support.
- You can keep your feet on the ground with knees bent or experiment with different leg positions. Try extending one or both legs out long to stretch the front body. Or lift one or both legs up in the air. You can move and stretch or hold them in place.

■ Stay in the pose for 5 to 20 minutes. You can change your leg position as many times as you like. When you're ready to come out of the posture, bring the soles of your feet to the floor and lift your hips to slide the bolster out from under you. Gently lower your hips to the floor. Rock your knees side to side to clear tension from your hips and low back.

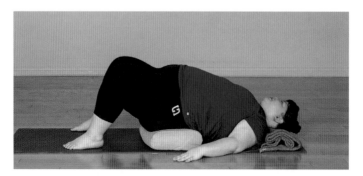

Figure 7.1   Supported bridge pose.

Pose Options

■ Experiment with different types and heights of support underneath you. Add one or more folded blankets to extend the height of your bolster. The higher the support, the more intense backbend and front-body stretch you can get.

■ Try different leg positions as you hold the pose. Bring both legs up and make a pedaling motion as if you were riding a bike. Or get more support by placing a strap around your feet and lifting the legs (see figure 7.2). Use the strap to hold some of the weight of your legs as you stretch and move. Or use the support to hold the weight of your legs as you keep them lifted and still. Get creative and explore all the options available to you in this position!

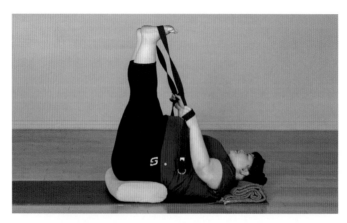

Figure 7.2   Supported bridge pose with the legs up and a strap supporting weight.

Accessible Challenges

▪ Switch the support under you to something with a firmer texture to provide a different experience. Try using one or more blocks under your hips (see figure 7.3). When using a block for support, make sure it's placed directly under your sacrum and not in the dip of your lower back. (Your sacrum is located below the dip of your lower back and above your buttocks.)

▪ Raise the height of the support under you to increase the amount of backbend and front-body stretch you get.

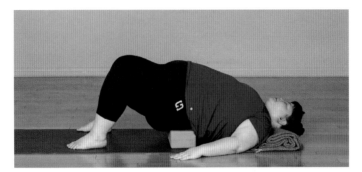

Figure 7.3   Supported bridge pose on blocks.

Tips for Plus-Sized Bodies

Some plus-sized folks have sensitivity on or around their sacrum, where the spine connects to the hips. It can be uncomfortable to use blocks to elevate the hips since blocks have a firmer texture and hard edges. Be sure to try the bolster option if you find you have sensitivity in that area. It can make supported bridge pose much more comfortable!

Legs-Up-the-Wall Pose (Viparita Karani)

This posture brings a gentle stretch of the legs and relief for back pain and headaches. It is amazing after a long day of sitting, walking, or traveling when your body is feeling stressed and tired. I often find myself coming into legs-up-the-wall when I'm feeling fatigued, my feet are hurting, or my ankles are swollen. It can be a relaxing way to find rejuvenation after many different activities. Be sure to adapt the pose to perfectly support your body. It can be performed on the floor against a wall as is traditional, as well as on the bed with your legs up a headboard, on the couch with your legs up the back support, on the floor with your legs up on a chair, and really any way you'd like to set it up. Find what works for you and your environment to make the pose your own!

Alignment Checklist

- Sit on the floor with your legs in front of you and the whole right side of your body touching the wall. Place your left hand on the floor behind and to the left of your body and start to lean your weight into your hand.

- As you lean into the hand, swing your legs up onto the wall and bring your shoulders and head gently down onto the floor. You want to end up lying on your back with your hips to the wall and your legs raised and resting on the wall. If you end up with your hips away from the wall, scoot your body forward until they come as close to the wall as possible. This might feel very strange. You might fall over. Don't worry, that's normal! Move slowly and be gentle and patient with yourself.

- Place your arms in a position that feels comfortable. You might try extending them overhead to rest on the floor or down by your sides.

- Engage your legs only as much as you need to keep them vertical and in place. You can rest a folded blanket on the soles of your feet and loop a strap around your calves to help keep your legs in place without using your muscles (see figure 7.4).

- Close your eyes or soften your gaze. Rest in the pose for 5 to 20 minutes. Cover yourself with a blanket to help promote feelings of comfort and safety. Place an eye pillow on your eyes to block the light and stimulate your vagus nerve to help you relax.

- To come out of the posture, let your legs slide down to the floor and come to lie on your side. Stay here for a few moments, release the strap if you're using it, and then slowly come up to a seated position.

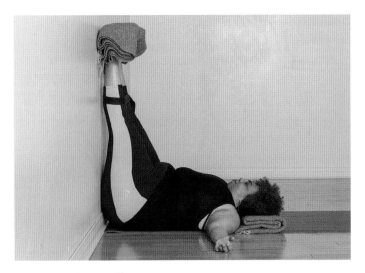

Figure 7.4   Legs-up-the-wall pose.

Pose Options

■ Experiment with leg positions to change how the pose feels. Make different shapes but keep your connection to the wall so the posture is fully supported. Try bringing the legs out into a wide V, soles of the feet together with your knees out to the sides, feet to the wall, and your knees to your chest, or anything you can think of.

■ Use what you have! Instead of putting your legs on the wall, try putting them on a chair seat (see figure 7.5), the back of a couch, the headboard of a bed, a coffee table or ottoman, and anywhere else you can find.

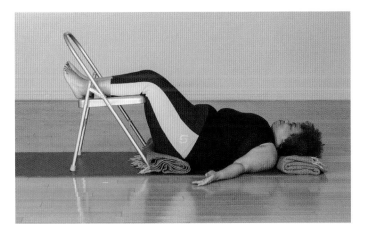

Figure 7.5   Legs-on-a-chair pose.

Accessible Challenges

Instead of bringing your hips to the floor or on a folded blanket, try creating a taller support. Place a bolster, stack of folded blankets, blocks, or another support under your hips.

Tips for Plus-Sized Bodies

For plus-sized folks who have sensitivity on or around their sacrum, it can be uncomfortable to elevate the legs and cause more pressure on that area in legs-up-the-wall. If you experience discomfort, add a folded blanket, a thin pillow, or a bolster under your sacrum to make the posture more comfortable so you can stay in it as long as you like.

Reclining Bound-Angle Pose (Supta Baddha Konasana)

A variation of the seated pose, reclining bound-angle is a hip-opening posture often performed on the floor with props to provide extra support. It can also be practiced while seated on a chair for a very similar result. Either way you practice it, reclining bound-angle pose can bring a gentle stretch to your inner thighs, hips, and knees. Many practitioners find the pose to be helpful in creating grounding and opening feelings in the body.

Alignment Checklist

■ Lie on your back with a folded blanket under your head if that is comfortable. Bring the soles of your feet together and angle your knees out to each side. You can place a block set at any height under each knee to get some support while you hold the pose (see figure 7.6).

■ Arrange your arms in any comfortable position. If it works for your body, try bringing your arms out to the sides or into a high V, palms turned up. Cover yourself with a blanket to help promote feelings of comfort and safety. Place an eye pillow on your eyes to block the light and stimulate your vagus nerve to help you relax.

■ Hold here for as long as it feels comfortable to you. In the beginning, you may find that shorter hold times are gentler on your body. Be kind to yourself and start slowly. You can always lengthen your hold time as you practice more.

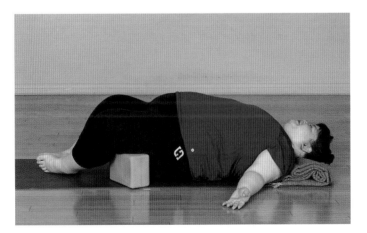

Figure 7.6   Reclining bound-angle pose.

Pose Options

Try the pose while seated in a chair (see figure 7.7). Sit on the chair with your back to the chair back for support. Place a bolster underneath your feet with soles together. You want to feel very supported here so your body can release tension. Roll a blanket into a long tube and place the middle around your neck with each end hanging down and tucked under your arms. Rest your head back on the blanket and soften into the posture.

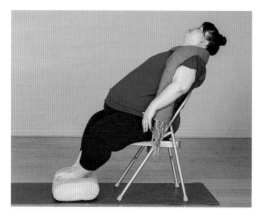

Figure 7.7   Bound-angle pose on a chair.

Accessible Challenges

■ Experiment with elevating your hips while you hold the position. Place a bolster underneath your hips, as in supported bridge pose, and follow the instructions for the reclining bound-angle pose.

■ Use a strap looped and secured around your waist and feet to hold your body in position (see figure 7.8). You can use the strap to hold your feet's natural position or you can tighten the strap to bring your feet closer toward your torso and hold them there without using your muscles.

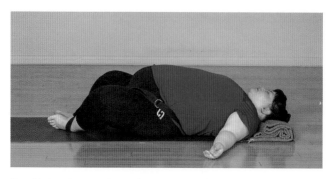

Figure 7.8   Reclining bound-angle pose with a strap.

Tips for Plus-Sized Bodies

In this, and any other reclined positions, practitioners with large breasts may find it more challenging to breathe. If this is the case for you, elevate your shoulders and head to change the angle of your body and make it easier and more comfortable to breathe.

Supported Fish Pose (Matsyasana)

Supported fish pose is a great stretch for the front of the body, which is particularly helpful for those of us who tend to slouch over our keyboards and phones all day. It can be very gentle but incredibly impactful for many folks. This is another posture I love to practice at the end of a long day. In fact, I often set myself up for the seated version while I'm still at my desk. It feels amazing after a long day of computer work! I can feel the fatigue and tightness in my body melt away, and it refreshes me for the rest of the evening.

Alignment Checklist

■ Roll a blanket into a short tube and place it widthwise across your mat. Lie on your back with the bottom of your shoulder blades resting on the rolled blanket. You may need to scoot yourself up or down the mat to get positioned correctly.

■ You want to end up with your shoulders on the mat and your chest lifted and stretching. Your head will be tilted so that your chin is lifted and the front of your throat is open (see figure 7.9).

■ Arrange your legs in any position that feels comfortable. Cover yourself with a blanket to help promote feelings of comfort and safety. Place an eye pillow on your eyes to block the light and stimulate your vagus nerve to help you relax.

■ Hold as long as feels good to you. If the pose feels intense, you may want to start with shorter hold times and work your way up.

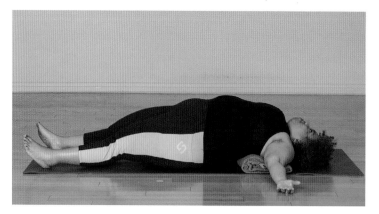

Figure 7.9 Supported fish pose.

Pose Options

■ You can adjust the intensity of the pose by rolling your blanket more to make the support taller or less to make the support shorter.

■ You can lessen the intensity of the stretch by placing some support underneath your head.

■ Try the pose while seated on a chair (see figure 7.10). Sit on the chair with your back to the chair back for support. Place a bolster widthwise behind the middle of your back and lean back into it. Make sure your feet are supported by the floor or blocks. Roll a blanket into a long tube and place the middle around your neck with each end hanging down and tucked under your arms. Rest your head back on the blanket and soften into the posture.

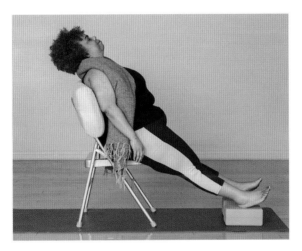

Figure 7.10   Supported fish pose on a chair.

Accessible Challenges

■ Add a hip-opening element by bringing the soles of your feet together and angling your knees out to each side.

■ Replace the blanket underneath you with blocks for a firmer support and higher lift of the chest.

Tips for Plus-Sized Bodies

Practitioners with large breasts may find it more challenging to breathe in this posture. If this is the case for you, try looping a strap around your chest and tightening it enough to keep your breasts in place. Be sure not to overtighten the strap and make breathing a challenge or cause discomfort. If a strap feels uncomfortable when used this way, you might benefit from using another type of prop that's specifically made to address this problem. Breast-support bands for yoga can be easily found online or at specialty retailers. These can be more comfortable than yoga straps, as can a tightly fitting sports bra or camisole.

Deep-Relaxation Pose (Savasana)

Some folks say they attend class only for the savasana at the end. I'm certainly a fan of the deep-relaxation pose, although other people find it to be the most difficult of all the postures! As a teacher, I can attest to the fact that many students struggle with stillness and being at rest. It can be very challenging to ask yourself to release the racing thoughts that occupy your mind throughout the day. This is exactly why we need the deep-relaxation pose at the end of class. It's the perfect time to give yourself a moment of calm to get centered before you leave and return to the rest of the world.

Don't be tempted to skip this pose! This part of your practice is so important that, if you have only a little time, I recommend selecting a couple postures to move the body and work out tension and then spend the remainder of your time in the deep-relaxation pose. The movement prepares your body for stillness, allowing you to release tension and feel refreshed. They work together to create a balanced practice and to give you all the benefits available!

Traditionally, deep-relaxation pose was practiced on the back, but there are tons of positions that can bring ease and relaxation into your body. Check the Pose Options section for ideas!

Alignment Checklist

- Lie on your back with your legs out long. Place a folded blanket or small pillow under your head for softness and support (see figure 7.11).

- Check in with your lower back and see if it feels relaxed or uncomfortable. If it's arching away from the floor, try placing a block under each knee or thigh. If it needs a higher support, replace the blocks with a bolster or even bring your legs to rest on a chair seat.

- Arrange your arms in the most comfortable position. Know that you can always change your position if you stop feeling comfortable. Cover yourself with a blanket to help promote feelings of comfort and safety. Place an eye pillow on your eyes to block the light and stimulate your vagus nerve to help you relax.

- Soften the muscles in your face, wiggle your jaw, and allow your tongue to rest against the roof of your mouth.

- Hold for 5 to 15 minutes or longer if you want. To come out of the pose, roll gently onto your right side. Stay here for a few breaths and then slowly bring yourself up to a seated position.

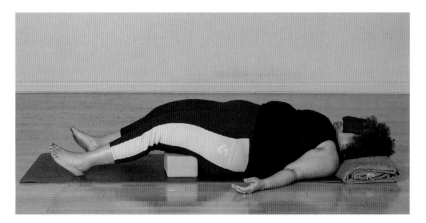

Figure 7.11 Deep-relaxation pose.

Pose Options

◻ Try the pose on your side, with something soft under your head and a folded blanket padding between your knees and feet (see figure 7.12*a*).

◻ Experience the deep-relaxation pose from a seated position on the floor (see figure 7.12*b*). Sit on a folded blanket with your legs out wide. Place a bolster vertically in front of you and tilt it toward you. Rest your head on top of the bolster and wrap your arms around it. You can turn your head either direction or rest your chin on the bolster.

◻ Practice the deep-relaxation pose from a seated position on a chair (see figure 7.12*c*). Sit with your back to the chair back for support. Make sure your feet are supported by the floor, blocks, or a bolster. Roll a blanket into a long tube and place the middle around your neck with each end hanging down and tucked under your arms. Rest your head back on the blanket and soften into the posture.

◻ Practice the deep-relaxation pose from a seated position on a chair, but with your legs elevated (see figure 7.12*d*). Sit with your back to the chair back for support. Bring your legs up onto the seat of a second chair. Your legs can be straight or bent with soles of the feet together. Roll a blanket into a long tube and place the middle around your neck with each end hanging down and tucked under your arms. Rest your head back on the blanket and soften into the posture.

◼ Try the pose from reclined on the floor with your legs resting on a chair seat (see figure 7.12e). Come to your back and bring your legs up to rest on the seat of a chair. Drape a blanket over yourself and tuck the end around your feet for support and warmth as you soften into the deep-relaxation pose. Don't forget to add a folded blanket or small pillow under your head and place an eye pillow on your eyes if you have one.

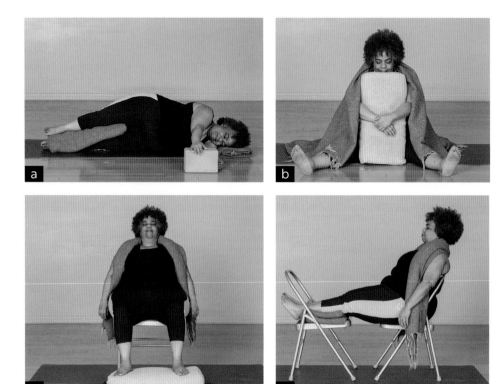

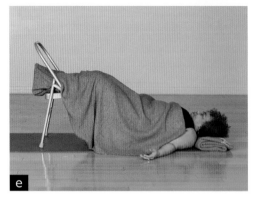

Figure 7.12 Deep-relaxation pose options: *(a)* on the side; *(b)* seated on the floor; *(c)* seated on a chair; *(d)* seated on a chair with legs elevated; *(e)* legs on a chair with blanket on top and tucked around feet.

Accessible Challenges

Add a breath work element by integrating one of the pranayama techniques in chapter 3 into the pose.

Tips for Plus-Sized Bodies

If lying on your back isn't working for your body, allow yourself to experiment with the side-lying and seated options. Just because the most taught version is supine, it doesn't mean that's the way you have to practice it!

CONCLUSION

Can you believe how many postures we've been through together? It's so exciting to learn about all the pose options, accessible challenges, and plus-size-specific tips that will make your practice completely customized to the needs of your body. We are through all the poses! Now you have a toolbox full of warm-up exercises and poses to take you through seated, kneeling, standing, reclined, and restorative elements of your practice.

How are you feeling after learning so much and getting so many details thrown at you? What does your body need? What about your mind? How can you care for yourself so that you're feeling strong, ready, and excited to keep moving forward with your exploration of yoga? This would be a great time for you to experiment with some different options of poses you feel drawn to. It would also be a wonderful time to journal about the thoughts and feelings that have come up as you've moved through the book. Be sure to practice self-care and honor the needs of your body and mind, whatever they are. Move on to the next chapter or take a break and come back later. What is your right next step?

Regardless of what you do next, I'm excited to tell you what's coming up in chapter 8 because I think it's where the real fun starts! Now that you've filled your yoga toolbox with poses, it's time to put them together and get creative with sequences as you build your home yoga practice. This is where you really get to address your particular needs and tailor your practices to your body and mind. This is honestly my favorite part of my home yoga practice. I love checking in with myself to see how I'm feeling physically and mentally and then figuring out what kind of practice is perfect for that moment. Don't be overwhelmed! I'm going to lead you through all of this, and, by the end of the chapter, you'll be feeling confident and ready to start your home practice!

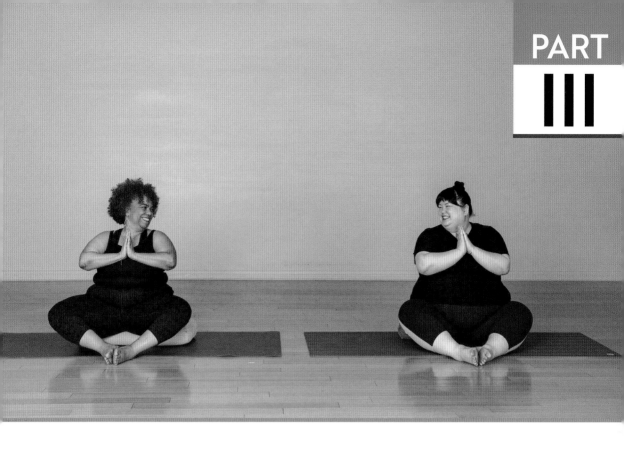

Make a Plan

CHAPTER 8

CREATING A HOME PRACTICE PLAN

If you ask yoga practitioners who have been practicing for decades if they have a secret to consistently hitting the mat and living their yoga practice, you will hear the same thing: Create a home practice that fits your needs and can be adjusted to any circumstance in your life. A strong home yoga practice is a powerful tool of self-care that can be your guide and friend through all of life's ups and downs.

I can attest to the power of a consistent home practice! It was the home yoga I did in conjunction with reading about body positivity that saved my life so many years ago. Learning to connect with my body that I had both ignored and punished with overexercise was the starting point to a new way of relating to and caring for my body.

It's hard though. Figuring out where to set up for your practice, what to do once you're on the mat, how to advocate for space and quiet, and everything else that comes along with a home yoga practice can feel incredibly overwhelming! But it's also really exciting. I'm so happy you have this book to be a resource for you as you create your own home practice. You get to create exactly the practice your body needs! Inside this chapter, you'll find information to help guide you through the process of figuring out what you need from a home practice. We'll tackle the myths I most commonly hear from my students when we talk about yoga at home. I'll give you some thought-provoking prompts to think about as you shape what your practice will become. We'll dive into the deep end and define the purpose of your practice in tangible terms that you can use to get started as you set up the space in your home and begin to create or find sequences to suit your personal needs.

First, let's start with some questions to mull over as you begin to think about your future home practice. We're all coming to this point with different experiences and needs, so it's helpful to get clear on them in the beginning. Start with basic questions: Why am I creating this home yoga practice? How will a home yoga practice enrich my life? What has stopped me from creating a home yoga practice up to this point? Examining the past for patterns and helpful information can guide the decisions you make next. Later in the chapter, we'll dig deeper into the specifics of what you need to get out of your practice, but, for now, try thinking more about the bigger picture in terms of what a home practice could do for you. What would it feel like to have a strong home practice? Also, think about any times when you've tried to start practicing yoga at home before, or maybe just thought about beginning and never made it past the planning phase. Whatever happened in the past, it's time to examine it and let go of any lingering bad vibes or feelings. If you've tried to start a practice before and it didn't work out, it doesn't mean the same thing will happen this time! Allow any thoughts or feelings to come up and to be acknowledged and then released. This is a blank slate for you to start fresh with the intentions and excitement you have in this moment.

COMMON MYTHS

Over the years, I've heard of countless myths and misconceptions from students and other yoga teachers about what a home yoga practice should look like, include, and strive for. It certainly feels like I've heard it all! If you find that any of the following myths resonate with you, know that you're not alone. Most folks go into the creation of a home yoga practice with ideas that are more harmful than helpful. These ideas keep us from starting what could be a beautiful and impactful personal practice because we fear that we won't do it right. What I hope you'll take away from this chapter is a feeling of freedom to try, to fail, to learn, and to grow. The ingrained ideas we have about what we need in order to start a home practice serve mostly to keep us frozen with fear and indecision. I know this is definitely true for me! I spent a long time thinking that I would start my home practice once I was ready to commit to intense and lengthy daily practices with all the props I could imagine in a picture-perfect yoga room. This way of thinking kept me from even trying to start a practice and deprived me of all those years I could have been enjoying the life-changing benefits of yoga. Take it from me, you have what you need, and you're ready right now. Let's do it!

Myth I: I Have to Practice Every Day for at Least an Hour and Do a Lot of Poses

Since standard studio yoga classes are usually an hour long, it's commonly assumed that home practices should be for the same length of time. I get it, really. It makes sense to model your practice after a studio class. However, in real life, you're not scheduling around other classes and trying to run your life like a studio. Your home practice doesn't need to be modeled after a studio class since the goals and needs are different. Your home practice might be a series of hour-long practices if that works best for you. Consider that your practices might look radically different than that. Before you decide how long your practices should be and how many poses to fit into that time frame, think about what you really want to get out of the time. It may be that your practices are mostly infrequent meditation sessions, daily breathing exercises, or occasional 20-minute flows to get your body moving after work.

Take a moment to release any expectations you have about starting a home yoga practice. Remember that your practices don't need to look like anyone else's, and you are free to create exactly what you need for each day.

Myth II: I Have to Go Hard, Sweat, and Really Push Myself

Western culture has created an attitude about yoga that lends itself to competition and comparison. One of the greatest gifts you could give yourself would be to release the need to compete with and compare yourself to others. Even taking on the attitude of competing with yourself can lead to harmful overexertion and missing out on the true benefits of yoga. If you've practiced yoga in a studio, it's highly possible that you encountered this competitive view of yoga already. Many studios market themselves in such a way that leads you to aspire to be like someone else, or even to want to be more than them. There is often a focus on pushing yourself hard, even to your breaking point, as a way of finding satisfaction and empowerment.

Yoga is not a competition between yourself and others, or even between you and your body and mind. Ask yourself if you are in the mood to find challenge, test your limits, and push yourself because it feels good or interesting to do so. What is your motivation for finding intensity on the mat? If the desire comes from a belief that you need to prove yourself or compete with others, it may be time to reevaluate your drive. Each time you practice, you have a choice of what to do, how long to do it, which postures to include, the type of breathing and meditation you'd like to experience, and any other aspect of your practice. Some days a calming, slow-flow practice is exactly what you need. Other times, your body is craving strong, powerful movement and deep-breathing exercises. Listening to your body is the only way to find that correct yoga practice for you. Remember to go inward to find inspiration for your home yoga practice. Honoring your mind and body's needs is the best way to choose your practice style.

Myth III: I Don't Have Room in My Home to Practice

We see some really beautiful yoga spaces on television and social media. I have often looked at those spaces and wished I had such a gorgeous and inspiring place to practice in. It's hard to see those amazing spaces in the media and then look around your own home for a place to practice with a grateful eye. Where is my bright and airy wall of windows? Where is my perfectly styled outdoor yoga cabana? All I have to work with is a patch of floor and my mat.

You know what? That's totally fine! I talk to so many people about starting a home yoga practice, and one of the most common things I hear is that they don't have enough room.

Personally, I think that anyone can find the space in their home to practice yoga. Whether you live in a tiny house or have eight roommates, lots of children, or more cats than you can count, you can find a solution for your practice. We'll talk in more detail about this later in the chapter, but, for now, just know that, if you want it to happen, you can do it. I have some great tips for carving out space in your home and setting emotional and physical boundaries with yourself and others. You can make this work!

Myth IV: I Need All New Equipment and Every Kind of Prop Before I Can Start

I don't know about you, but I often approach a new interest with the urge to buy every single material, component, recommended book, and helpful tool before I allow myself to even begin the hobby or practice. I've heard from tons of folks who have the same feeling as me, even about yoga. Perhaps, even especially about yoga! We decide that we can't start to practice until we have a new mat, blocks, special yoga blankets, a strap, videos or a streaming service membership, and anything else that we see other yoga practitioners using on social media. I get it! I have a craft cabinet loaded with full sets of tools and supplies for a number of different crafts. Did I need all the tools for bookbinding before I even tried it out? Absolutely not. Do you need all the yoga props before you even start to practice? Absolutely not.

I completely understand the desire to load up your cart with all the yoga stuff you think you need, and I encourage you to examine your impulse. For many of us, the urge to buy all the tools stems from excitement and a desire to be prepared. For others, it's a sign that we are nervous about the new endeavor and looking at our purchases as a means to help us feel ready. Sometimes, a gentle look at our motivation is the best thing we can do for ourselves. It's one thing to be prepared for your new home practice, but you don't need to put off getting started because you don't have all the props you might want.

Props are wonderful things! I think we've established by now that I am in love with yoga props and the accessibility they bring. However, a nonslip surface and some homemade or repurposed home accessories can go a long way in your yoga practice. Remember that a lap blanket from your couch, a dog leash, a stack of books duct-taped together, and lots of other creatively used items can get you started and work just fine until you decide if you want to purchase permanent versions. Don't let yourself put off getting the benefits of yoga because you don't have blocks yet.

Myth V: I Can't Try Yoga Until I Lose Weight

As plus-sized folks, we sometimes have the tendency to put things off until our circumstances are different, often when we lose weight. This is something I've experienced myself and heard from countless folks over the years. We decide that the thing we really want to do is not possible for us until we change our bodies or lives in some way. We think we don't deserve to have or experience the things that thinner people do. I get it! I really, really do. I've been there and felt those things deeply in my heart. What I've learned over time is that we're wrong. I hope you hear me when I say that you deserve to take the trip, try the trend, and put yourself out there no matter what size your body is. You deserve to live your life now. The body you have right now deserves to experience the joy of movement and the wonderful benefits that a yoga practice can bring.

DEFINE YOUR PURPOSE

We all come to yoga with different needs, inspirations, and intentions. When it comes to developing a strong home practice, you may be looking for increased embodiment and grounding, energy and an effective mood booster to start your mornings, or gentle strength-building exercises to complement your other activities. You may also be unsure of what exactly you want out of your practice, and that's ok! Many people come to yoga with a vague notion of feeling better, being more connected to themselves, or making an impact on their mental and physical health. If you don't know exactly what you want out of your practice, you can figure it out along the way.

I have some questions I like to ask folks who come to me for help starting their home practice:

■ What does it mean to listen to your body? What thoughts come up when you start to listen to your body's needs?

■ How do you want your practice to make you feel, physically and emotionally?

■ What goals do you have that yoga could help you achieve?

Consider these questions and reflect on the answers that come to mind. You can even use the questions as journaling prompts if that appeals to you. Before going through the questions, take a few deep, clearing breaths and give yourself permission to be open and honest with yourself.

Listening to your body is a hugely important part of your yoga practice, but it's something that is challenging and even scary for many people. As plus-sized folks, we can sometimes be especially out of practice at listening to our bodies since many of us spend years ignoring our needs and desires while we pursue unhealthy diets in an attempt to meet unrealistic expectations of beauty and body size. If you find yourself having a hard time connecting with your body and listening to what it needs or keep experiencing negative thoughts, please remember to be gentle with yourself.

Much of the healing work of yoga is about connecting with your body, being present, and learning to listen to your true needs and desires. As you ask yourself the previously mentioned questions, it may feel overwhelming. Give yourself permission to go slowly and to be as gentle with yourself as you would be with your closest friend or your child. Consider that your inner child deserves all the kindness you reserve for others.

I often ask myself these questions so I can stay connected with my needs and desires. The answers change! Sometimes, I ask myself and hear that I want to feel comforted and nurtured emotionally and strong and grounded physically. Other times, my body tells me that I need to focus on being open and vulnerable emotionally and find flow and energy physically. Sometimes, I even think I know what my body needs and wants, and then I check in and am totally wrong! It's easy to think you know what you need when in reality you've spent decades ignoring your needs and listening to what others tell you about your body.

You are the expert on your body! Only you know what you need and what your personal goals should be. Ask yourself to be open and honest about what you would like to accomplish with your yoga practice. Do you want to improve your cardiovascular system, gain flexibility, find strength, heal from an injury, increase your stamina, connect with your body in a meaningful way, learn to meditate, or boost your mood? Maybe your goal is different than anything I mentioned here. You can create your home practice to support whatever it is you're hoping to achieve. Remember that goals can change over time, so checking in with yourself regularly is a helpful activity.

WHEN TO PRACTICE

Depending on your needs, goals, and schedule, you may decide that a morning, afternoon, or evening practice is best for you. Figuring this out is important for creating the best possible practice, so take your time thinking through your needs and time commitments. Where do you have room in your schedule to add in a practice? Does the available time match your needs? Are you a morning person who would like to capitalize on that characteristic by practicing energizing yoga to start your day? Or consider an afternoon practice that could help you transition from work to home and give you some extra energy in the evenings. Many folks use a calming meditation and gentle yoga practice before bed to prepare their bodies for a good night's sleep. Consider whether your schedule can accommodate the type of practice that would benefit you most. If not, think about how you can make space in your day for your practice.

I would also encourage you to think about your practice as something that can happen throughout your day. Instead of a set time to step on your mat, your day might benefit from weaving in postures, breathing exercises, and meditation between your activities. I love to wake up and do gentle poses while still in bed, use the kitchen counters as a support to move and stretch more while I wait for the coffee to brew, take breaks during the workday to practice a few desk yoga poses, engage in calming breath work in the car, and meditate before bed. I don't do everything every day, but I do intersperse all of it throughout the week to keep me feeling grounded and centered. Some weeks, I don't step on the mat for a personal practice at all! During those weeks, I count on my little bits here and there to get me through. Very few people have the time and capacity to step on the mat every single day and practice for any great length of time. I recommend figuring out what your purpose is so you can decide when the best time is for you to practice. You may find that you're like me and decide to weave yoga into every day in small ways.

HOW TO PRACTICE

I discussed some of the styles of yoga in chapter 1, and I encourage you to take another look to refresh your memory before you continue with this section. The most popular styles of yoga that you find at studios in the United States are very different from each other. While some people find one style they like and stick with that, there are many who call on multiple styles to give them the benefits they're looking for. I teach hatha yoga, which is a personal favorite of mine for its gentle and slower approach to coming into and out of poses. At home in my personal practice, I often use hatha yoga as a base for the postures and then add in vinyasa, or flow yoga, because it feels nice in my body. I love to mix in different styles to bring variety to my home yoga. Restorative poses add calming, yin pose techniques allow me to deeply stretch and focus on alignment with support, and power yoga sequences give me the challenge I'm looking for when I'm in the mood to sweat it out on the mat.

It'll take time for you to experiment with different styles of yoga and find what your body needs. The best thing you can do is allow yourself to be curious and adventurous and to take safe risks! Give yourself permission to be open and vulnerable and try new styles. You might hate them, and that's okay. No one likes everything. Encourage the curiosity that lives inside of you, and you might find some new styles of yoga, wellness tips, or even friends that you never expected. Remember that you deserve to live your life fully right now. The best yoga practices are diverse and always changing as we learn and grow over time.

As you explore the different types of yoga and their benefits, you may find that there are needs your body has that props can fulfill. I wrote about props in chapter 2, and I mentioned a ton of options for a practice. You definitely don't need to have everything on that list; even I don't! However, as you try various kinds of yoga, keep an eye out for props that might make the experience better. For example, in a yin yoga class, we use blocks, blankets, bolsters, and straps to support our bodies so we can hold a pose for a long time. If you find yourself drawn to yin yoga, you might want to DIY or purchase some of these props to enhance your practice. The same can be said for any style of yoga. Power yoga practitioners often invest in extra sticky mats and superabsorbent towels because the practice tends to make you sweat a lot. Restorative yoga uses even more props than yin yoga, so, if you love the restorative practices, you'll probably want to gather multiples of bolsters, blankets, blocks, sandbags, and straps.

Depending on what styles of yoga you come to love to practice, you'll want to slowly start to grow your collection of props that help you have the best possible experience. Remember that the goal of using props is not to get to the point where you don't need them anymore. The goal of using props is to support the body, to find accessible challenges, and to experience the postures in new and interesting ways. I hear from some people who don't want to make or purchase any props because they believe they won't need them for long. I firmly encourage you to invest your energy or money into the props that would fit best into your practice. They are your helpers in keeping your practice fresh, fun, and safe!

SET YOUR SPACE

No matter what circumstances you're working with at your home, the space around you makes an impact on your mood, focus, and, ultimately, the quality of your yoga practice. This section explores how to create an intentional yoga space in your home that feels authentic to you and sets you up for a great practice. We'll begin by thinking about how much space you really need and then tackle some of the challenges you face in your home. Let's examine qualities of a space that are important to you and help you come up with options to make your environment feel and function the best it can.

Find the Right Space

It's common for folks to decide a home practice isn't for them because they think they don't have enough room. We see ideal yoga spaces presented to us as typical on television, in movies, and on social media. While it would be wonderful to have a whole room full of light, plants, and perfectly coordinated yoga accessories to ourselves just for practicing yoga, that's not reality for most of us. Many of us live in spaces where the only unclaimed expanse of floor is part of a walkway, by a bed, or in the kitchen. That's okay! Your yoga practice doesn't need a whole room to itself, it doesn't need complete privacy, and it certainly doesn't need to be picture perfect. Your yoga practice is just that— yours. If you have access to a private space that you can turn into a permanent yoga space, awesome! If not, it's fine to use whatever space you can to the best of your ability. If that means unrolling your yoga mat in the kitchen, so be it! Let's explore the components of a great yoga space and then get you off on your own to get your hands dirty and create your space.

Think about your home and ask yourself if you have a room, nook, or other area that you can permanently dedicate to your yoga practice. This might include a guest room, a corner or other section of a shared space like a living room, or even an outdoor space if you live somewhere with amenable weather. If you don't, where can you find space in your home to unroll your mat and stretch your arms and legs out in most directions? Don't worry about being able to decorate or embellish the space right now. We'll discuss how to plan for portable decorations later. For now, think about the spaces you've identified and narrow the options down based on how private, comfortable, and appealing they are to you. Consider what is important to you about your yoga space and choose the one that ticks the most boxes off your list. Take into account the presence of windows, a comfortable temperature, and anything else that feels like a priority to you.

Some spaces are permanent areas that can be dedicated to your yoga practice at all times. This means you can decorate however you like and leave all your yoga accessories out without worrying about them getting moved, ruined, or being in the way. Other spaces are temporary spaces, which means you'll be able to use them for your yoga practice and then need to put everything away after you're finished. Regardless of the space being permanent or temporary, there are positive attributes that have led you to choose it. Think through all those positive elements and list them to yourself. Be sure to think about things like access to natural light, storage or space to store props, plants, amount of foot traffic to contend with, noise level, etc. Think through all the good things about the space that come to mind. What are the drawbacks to the space? Think about the space's challenges that you'll want to address so you can be ready to come up with solutions later.

Make the Space Feel Special and Intentional

Take a moment to think about your home decor style and how your ideal yoga aesthetic fits into it. What kind of decorations speak to your soul and make you feel the way you want your yoga practice to make you feel? Many articles on creating a home yoga space will encourage you to use minimalist decor and light colors, but if that's not your personal style, it's not the right thing to do. You want your yoga space to feel authentically you, and if that means dark, moody colors and lots of art, so be it! Think about your favorite spaces you've seen and what they have in common. Ask yourself how you want to feel in your yoga space and then think about the colors, design aesthetics, and types of decorations that align with that feeling. Don't worry if your home doesn't already have those things. Allow yourself to be creative and get your design ideas flowing. If you'd like, you can make notes about aesthetics, designs, colors, and energy. Or mull it over and keep everything in your mind. This is all about you, so feel free to process in the best way for your brain.

Then, consider the space you're working with and what is possible. If your space is not permanently used for yoga, you'll need to find or create storage space nearby for props and decorations. Are there cabinets, drawers, or storage baskets nearby that can be repurposed to hold your yoga supplies? Is there space on the wall to add a shelf or other storage unit? How can you use the resources available to highlight and enhance the positive characteristics of your space? For example, if the space you've chosen has great natural light, you might think of ways to highlight the window or door by hanging curtains or cleaning the glass, facing that direction for your practice, or simply opening the blinds or curtains to let in the most light possible. If there is room on the wall or in other surrounding areas to add some decorative elements, think about the colors and textures that appeal to you and would support the mood and energy you're wanting to bring into your practice. Can you store your props in a basket, box, or cabinet that you love? Find items from around your home that you can repurpose into decoration for your yoga space. If you can leave them there all the time, that's great. If not, find a box or other container to use as the vehicle for all your supplies so it's easy to set up and pack away the items you want for your practice. If you make it easy to prepare your space, you're more likely to actually practice!

Create Boundaries to Hold Your Space as Sacred

A lot of the challenge folks face with their yoga space is not even about the actual space itself. For many, it's about how to hold the space they're in and their time on the mat as sacred for themselves. Depending on your living situation, you may have challenges with setting and enforcing physical or emotional boundaries with roommates, partners, children, and even yourself. If you have your own room permanently dedicated to yoga, live alone, and can focus easily on your practice, this part can be much easier. Having access to a permanent and private room provides built-in physical boundaries that can help to keep your space and time sacred for you. If you have a semiprivate permanent or temporary yoga space, you may need to change things up around you to create that sacred space. Think of rearranging furniture to create physical boundaries and define your space. You can use large plants, lamps, curtains, and other furniture and decorations from around your home to create these boundaries for your space. Often, simply defining the space works to remind others in the home that they should wait to talk to you until you're finished with your practice. These physical boundaries also help you to focus on yourself and your practice instead of getting caught up in what's happening around you.

Think about what you can do in your space to define it and claim it as your sacred area. It might help to also speak to the other occupants of your home about what might help them remember to hold their conversation or questions until after your practice is over. Sometimes people will think of things they find helpful that you'd never think of yourself. This is especially useful when helping children understand why it's important to give you the space and time for your practice. Regardless of their age, involving the other people in the solution helps them to feel ownership of the situation. I've heard great feedback from folks who engaged their roommates, children, and partners in the process of creating these physical and emotional boundaries. If you have your own private room, the creation and enforcement of emotional boundaries may be easier, but not necessarily. Creating emotional boundaries requires you to work with your space sharers in order to hold your practice sacred. If you live with adults or children who don't respect closed doors or requests for alone and quiet time, you may spend a great deal of time reinforcing your boundaries even with a private space.

Regardless of whether your space is private, semiprivate, permanent, or temporary, boundaries are important! This is true even if you live alone. Part of setting these boundaries is getting clear with yourself about what you use the space for and what you are willing to allow in the space. For example, you might set boundaries with yourself about checking your social media, the Internet, or text messages. Or you may find it helpful to create boundaries with yourself around what kind of thoughts and energy you allow in the space. Many of us come to yoga to find compassion and love for ourselves and our bodies, and setting boundaries about negative self-talk can be empowering. Take some time to think about some boundaries you may need to set with others and with yourself.

Then, it's finally time to begin putting it all together! Regardless of whether it's a permanent or temporary space, you can experiment with different decorations and storage solutions for your mat and props to make it really feel sacred. Be mindful to stay true to what feels right for your space and practice. Don't worry about what yoga spaces look like in magazines or on social media. What's important here is that your yoga space works for your needs and aesthetic. You can always make changes to your space later, so try not to aim for perfection. Instead, focus on creating a space that feels nice to be in and is functional for what you want to get out of your practice. You can always tailor it to your specific needs once you have been practicing and have a better idea of what you need. Right now, your space doesn't have to be the perfect incarnation; it just has to be the right space for right now.

CREATE SEQUENCES THAT WORK FOR YOU

Let's talk about sequencing! What is a sequence and why is it important in yoga? How can you create sequences that can enhance your practice and support your body's needs and goals? I'll start with the definition of a sequence, which is simply the combination of poses, breath work, meditation, stretching, and whatever else you want in your home practice. You take these elements and put them in order to create sequences that bring the benefits you need. Sequences can be designed to feel energizing, calming, grounding, and affirming or to bring certain feelings and energy into your day. This section should help you learn about the different elements of a sequence and how to put them together to build a practice that works for your body. You may find that you want to have a couple different types of sequences at the ready for whatever your mood calls for. With practice and experimentation, you'll build a library of sequences to fit every mood and desire.

Depending on your goal, intention, and mood, you'll want to choose a style of yoga that delivers the right benefits. We discussed some popular types of yoga earlier in this chapter and in chapter 1. Take a peek to refresh your memory if that would be helpful. The first step to designing a sequence for yourself is to figure out the most basic goals for the practice. If you're looking to de-stress, ground yourself, or prepare for bed, then a restorative or yin yoga practice might be best. Conversely, if you want to energize yourself and get moving to start your day, you'll probably want to practice in the style of hatha or vinyasa yoga. If you'd like some examples of sequences to bring certain types of energy into your day, check out chapter 9 for some great examples and full sequences to follow.

Elements of a Sequence

If you build your sequences with the following elements, you can be sure that you're covering your bases. The elements listed here are basic building blocks of yoga sequences. Once you're familiar with these, you'll be able to easily design all kinds of sequences to fit your mood and needs. Use these elements as a starting point for your yoga sequences but know that you can omit or add to these as you wish. There are no rules here! Experiment with these elements and see how you can tailor them for your practices.

Part I of the Sequence: Warm-Up

Warm-up postures, stretches, and breath work can be done from a standing, seated, or reclined position. The goal of the warm-up is to prepare your body for what is to come. Even very gentle practices such as a restorative sequence or a meditation and breath work practice need a warm-up. Sometimes the warm-up is less about warming the muscles and more about grounding and centering yourself to prepare your mind. Historically, the postures in yoga existed to prepare the body for meditation. It's much easier for a body to be in stillness when it has had a chance to move and stretch beforehand.

Part II of the Sequence: Core of the Practice

This is the middle of your sequence. Your body is warmed up and ready for more movement. Try to make a progression of poses that continues to prepare your body for what comes next. Think about the postures coming up that will require certain areas to be properly prepared to prevent injury. Add in preparation poses to the beginning of the core of your practice so that the postures that come later can be performed safely. This kind of planning will get easier in time as you learn which postures are especially good at prepping for other poses.

Part III of the Sequence: Cool-Down

Cool-down postures, stretches, and breath work can be done from a standing, seated, or reclined position. The goal of the cool-down is to bring your breath and temperature down while performing poses and stretches that give your muscles what they need. Stopping abruptly without cooling down can lead to injury and soreness. Take the time to ease your way out of the more intense part of your practice. This gentle decrease in intensity is a kinder way to end your practice.

Part IV of the Sequence: Savasana

Savasana is the last step in your practice. It is a deep-relaxation pose that gives you time to reconnect with your breath, find ease in your body, and prepare to transition back into your day. This is your chance to find the most comfortable position possible, close your eyes, and release any tension in your body. For some, this is the best part of their practice, but, for others, it is very challenging. Savasana asks you to release control over your breath, relax your muscles, and allow your mind to let go of control over your thoughts. Don't skip this part of your practice! This element of your sequence is important because it gives you time to transition back into your day with ease and relaxation.

Put It All Together

All that's left is to add actual poses to your sequence! There are different ways to choose which postures to include in your practice. You can carefully plan them out, going into your practice with a solid idea of what you'll do, for how long, and with a specific goal in mind. You can also begin with a loose idea of a certain type of pose you want to include (hip opening, back stretching, etc.) and then let your body guide you to decide which specific poses to do. Work with your personality and do what feels natural for you. If you're someone who likes to have a plan mapped out, then follow your intuition! If you like to go with the flow and see what happens, honor that!

Generally, folks like to use one or more of the following ways to choose the poses for their practice. Feel free to try all of these and see which ones you like the most. It's common to find a couple of ways you enjoy the best and stick to those, but you are the boss!

Pose Cards

Yoga card decks have become a popular resource for yogis of all experience levels. These yoga decks are similar in size and material to playing cards, but, instead of numbers, each card has a pose on it. You can use these decks to choose random poses to add to your sequence or lay them out and select the postures intentionally. The great thing about these decks is that they are portable and easy to use.

Intuitive Flowing

For those who want to connect with their bodies and practice listening and intuitive movement, this kind of unplanned flowing might be a great tool. With intuitive flowing, you simply start your practice with some basic poses and see where your body takes you. This is a great way to keep your practice fresh since you'll probably move through a different mix of postures each time. If you like structure and planning out your sequence beforehand, this may be a challenging way to design your practice.

Sequences Designed by Others

Using sequences created by other people is a nice way to begin your practice easily if you are overwhelmed by the idea of designing your own. I love to use other people's sequences whether they're written or I'm following along to a recorded video. I recommend using other people's sequences to help you get familiar with new styles of yoga. It can be really helpful to experience the new style through an established sequence created by someone more familiar than yourself.

Set a Sequence That You Follow Again and Again

Some forms of yoga are practiced by repeating the same sequence every time you practice. Many people find it appealing to follow the same sequence each time as a form of moving meditation. I have a few sequences I follow when I want to move my body in certain ways or bring about particular types of energy. It can be very comforting to practice a sequence that you've done many times before.

Be adventurous and try out as many different types of sequences and forms of yoga as you can. Notice how it feels to practice each time and take note of what you liked, what you disliked, and how you would change it for the future. Write your notes in one place so you can easily remember your impressions and thoughts about each sequence and type of yoga. In time, you'll learn what your body likes best and what feels most natural for you.

CONCLUSION

I'd like to finish this chapter with a question I think is key to everyone's yoga practice, regardless of their goals and needs: What is the least you could do? Every day is different, and it's impossible to hold yourself to the same standard in every situation. When you're busy and overwhelmed and possibly starting to be unkind toward yourself, I want you to remember this question. What is the least you could do in this moment?

If stepping on the mat is not possible and you have very little time or capacity to practice the physical side of yoga, ask yourself this question: In this very moment, what is the tiniest yoga practice I could engage in? Could I set an intention for the rest of my day, take five deep breaths, stand barefoot in the grass and ground myself, sit in savasana for five minutes, or simply stand in mountain pose and feel my breath move through me? The least you can do is not something to scoff at! The least you can do is a powerful act of self-care in a moment when it would be easy to forgo it. You deserve to take that 30 seconds or five minutes or whatever you can spare and give yourself permission to do the least.

If you need some inspiration or a blueprint to follow, check out the next couple of chapters to get ideas or exact sequences to follow. Coming up in chapter 9 are energizing practices, which can be great tools to pump you up and get you through the day when your energy or spirit is flagging. I've included different lengths of practices so that you can fit it in no matter what else is going on. Remember that you don't have to follow these sequences, do the whole thing, or go in order. Check out the practices and see if any spark your motivation to hit the mat. Follow them exactly or use them as a springboard to experiment with the postures in your toolbox. There are so many possibilities. Give yourself permission to play!

CHAPTER 9

ENERGIZING PRACTICES

Sometimes we all feel tired, sluggish, or fatigued for various reasons. When this occurs, ask yourself what you need at that moment. Would resting be the best thing for your body and mind? Or would bringing in fresh energy and invigorating your body be the most helpful? If it's the latter, an energizing yoga practice might be just the thing to turn your day around. While most poses can be energizing to the body and mind, there are certainly some that work better than others for most folks. This chapter presents a number of sequences of varying lengths that I created to bring more energy into your day. The poses included are all explained in this book, so look out for the page numbers to refresh your memory about the benefits, alignment checklists, pose options, accessible challenges, and plus-size-specific tips.

During your practice, consider that it's not just the poses that you do, but it's the energy and intention you put into them. Think of mindfully performing them with enthusiasm and commitment. Use strong arms, engaged muscles, and bold movements. Focus on the sensations in your body and how your breath and energy move through you. Take big breaths when you need to. The energy you put into your practice helps to bring more energy into your body and mind. Take a look at the sequences included in this chapter to find what fits your needs best right now. There are sequences of different lengths and also options for a floor-based practice. Listen to your body's needs and remember to always honor what you hear.

Energizing Sequence I: 10 Minutes

This seated practice is a 10-minute sequence to bring fresh energy into your body. It's a great way to start your day or to shake off the afternoon slump that sometimes happens. Feel free to perform the sequence once or repeat it a few times for a longer practice if that feels right for you. All poses in this sequence are seated or kneeling, and you have the option of using a chair for support if kneeling doesn't work for your body.

Props Needed

Blanket

Chair

Blocks

Kneepad

Tips for Plus-Sized Bodies

Step wider or move the belly to make space in these postures. Place a kneepad or folded blanket under your knee in the lunge.

Pose	Photo	Pose notes	Pose options	Page
Bound-angle		Begin with three deep, clearing breaths. Focus on grounding yourself and getting present in your body. Hold for 6 to 10 breaths.	If your hips or back are uncomfortable, you can adjust your legs to any seated position.	63
Five-pointed star		Focus on extending out in all directions. Consider adding cat–cow pose, page 67, for spinal movement as you hold the pose for 10 breaths.	Bring your palms together and extend energetically out through your elbows if your shoulders feel stressed with arms out to the sides. Practice this pose from seated on the floor or on a chair.	105
Tabletop		Gently move your hips side to side or experiment with any kind of movement that feels interesting. Hold the pose for 10 breaths.	If your wrists are uncomfortable, come to a standing version of the pose with your hands on a chair seat.	65
Downward-facing dog		Raise and lower your heels or bend and straighten your knees. Hold for 8 to 10 breaths.	Keep your hands on the floor, on blocks, or on a chair seat.	96
Low-lunge and Half-monkey		Hold each pose for four to six breaths on each side.	Perform the standing version on a chair if kneeling is uncomfortable.	80 and 82

Energizing Sequence II: 30 Minutes

This seated practice is a 30-minute sequence to be performed from seated on the floor or on a chair for stability, support, and a fresh perspective on poses. The sequence can help to lift your mood and bring new energy into your day. It's a great evening practice for after work to elevate your energy and get your body moving after being at a desk or on your feet all day. Feel free to perform the sequence once or repeat it for a longer practice if that feels right for you. Many poses in this sequence can also be practiced from standing with a chair for support.

Props Needed

Chair

Tips for Plus-Sized Bodies

Step your feet wide and bring your belly to the center to make space in the forward-folds.

Pose	Photo	Pose notes	Pose options	Page
Mountain		Take six deep breaths. Focus on grounding yourself and getting present in your body.	Inhale and raise your arms overhead. Exhale and lower your arms by your sides.	91
Forward-fold		Repeat eight times, holding in the folded position for two to three breaths.	Widen your stance to make space for your belly.	49
Cat–cow		Move with your breath between cat and cow pose. Repeat eight times.	Practice from a standing position with your hands on the chair seat to mimic the alignment of the kneeling version.	67
Simple twist		Exhale into the twist and hold for six breaths on each side. Repeat four times.	Practice this pose from seated on the floor or on a chair.	70
Chair		Hold for six breaths and repeat four times. Choose any arm position that feels good.	Practice from a standing position or add a twist of the torso for an accessible challenge.	102

(continued)

Energizing Sequence II: 30 Minutes *(continued)*

Pose	Photo	Pose notes	Pose options	Page
Gate		Exhale into the posture and hold for 8 to 10 breaths. Repeat on each side two times.	Keep your chest turned toward the front.	74
Downward-facing dog		Raise and lower your heels or bend and straighten your knees. Hold for 8 to 10 breaths.	Keep your hands on the floor, on blocks, or on a chair seat.	96
Plank		Bring your hands to the chair seat and lower your hips to make a straight line from head to toe.	Move to a wall for a more supported option. Move to the floor, with or without support, for an accessible challenge.	86
Five-pointed star		Focus on extending out in all directions. Hold the pose for 10 breaths.	Practice from a standing position for an accessible challenge.	105
Cat–cow		Move with your breath between cat and cow pose. Repeat eight times.	Practice from a standing position with your hands on the chair seat to mimic the alignment of the kneeling version.	67
Forward-fold		Repeat eight times, holding in the folded position for two to three breaths.	Widen your stance to make space for your belly.	49
Mountain		Take six deep breaths. Focus on noticing the sensations in your body and connecting with your breath.	Inhale and raise your arms overhead. Exhale and lower your arms by your sides.	91
Savasana		Relax your breath and body. Hold for three to five minutes.	Practice from a seated or supine position. Use your props to make yourself comfortable.	152

Energizing Sequence III: 60 Minutes

This is a 60-minute sequence you can use when you need to bring more energy into your body and mind. The poses can be performed from a standing position, and there are options for using a chair for added stability, support, and a fresh perspective on poses. This longer sequence can bring some fresh new energy into your day and lighten your mood. It's an especially great way to start your day with high energy before work or brunch on the weekend.

Props Needed

Chair   Blocks

Strap   Blanket

Tips for Plus-Sized Bodies

Move your belly to create space in many of these poses. Extend the length of your arms with blocks or a strap.

Pose	Photo	Pose notes	Pose options	Page
Bound-angle		Begin with three deep, clearing breaths. Focus on grounding yourself and getting present in your body. Hold for 6 to 10 breaths.	Sit up on a folded blanket to make sitting on the floor more comfortable.	63
Cat–cow		Move with your breath between cat and cow pose. Repeat 10 times.	Come to tabletop, page 65, and practice from kneeling for an accessible challenge.	67
Simple twist		Exhale into the twist and hold for six to eight breaths on each side. Repeat two times.	Add dynamic movement by moving in and out of the twist with each inhale and exhale instead of holding the pose.	70
Wide-leg forward-fold		Exhale in the fold and hold for 10 breaths. Repeat three times.	Move your belly to the center to find a deeper stretch. Flex your feet to increase the stretch in your inner thighs.	78

(continued)

Energizing Sequence III: 60 Minutes *(continued)*

Pose	Photo	Pose notes	Pose options	Page
Head-to-knee		Hold the posture for 8 to 10 breaths. Repeat two times on each side.	Make sure your hips are facing the front. Sometimes they shift when getting into the pose.	76
Tabletop		Gently move your hips side to side or experiment with any kind of movement that feels interesting. Hold the pose for 10 breaths.	If your wrists are uncomfortable, come to a standing version of the pose with your hands on a chair seat.	65
Camel		Come into the pose and find the level of support you need. Tuck your toes under or place a bolster on your legs to give your hands support.	Place a pad or folded blanket under your knees to soften the ground. Practice the seated version in a chair if kneeling doesn't feel safe for your body.	72
Downward-facing dog		Hold for 8 to 10 breaths, lifting your heels one at a time and shifting your hips side to side and then come to standing.	Keep your hands on the floor, on blocks, or bring to a chair seat. Stay here longer if it feels particularly good.	96
Mountain		Take six deep breaths and focus on the sensations in your body. Play with lifting your heels and adding a balance element to the pose.	Roll a blanket and place it under your heels to lift them with support. Experiment with closing your eyes as you lift and lower your heels for an accessible challenge.	91
Extended side-angle		Hold the posture for 8 to 10 breaths on each side. Repeat two times.	Bring your hand to a chair seat for a taller and more stable support. Lift your bottom arm up for an accessible challenge.	110
Warrior II		Hold for six breaths on each side. Repeat two times.	Practice from seated on a chair for more support. Add in five-pointed star, page 105, between each side for an accessible challenge.	113
Forward-fold		Repeat four times, holding in the folded position for two to three breaths. Practice with a wider stance if you prefer.	Step your feet wider apart, and come into deep-squat, page 115, for an accessible challenge.	94

Pose	Photo	Pose notes	Pose options	Page
Downward-facing dog		Raise and lower your heels or bend and straighten your knees. Hold for 8 to 10 breaths.	Keep your hands on the floor, on blocks, or on a chair seat.	96
Tabletop		Exhale into the pose and hold for 10 breaths. Move your torso forward and back and your hips side to side.	Step feet back into plank, page 86, and hold for an accessible challenge.	65
Low-lunge and Half-monkey		Come into each pose and hold for six breaths on each side. Repeat two times.	Place a pad under your knees and bring your hands to blocks or a chair seat. Practice these poses from a standing position with your foot on a chair seat if kneeling is uncomfortable.	80 and 82
Sphinx		Inhale up into the backbend and exhale back down. Move with your breath for six breaths. Come up and hold for as long as it feels like a challenge for you.	Practice cobra, page 127, in addition to sphinx for an accessible challenge. Come to standing and perform the pose on a wall for a different experience or if lying belly down is uncomfortable.	124
Supported bridge		Come into the pose and hold for 20 breaths or as long as you like.	Blocks will give a firmer support but can be uncomfortable for some. Try a bolster underneath instead.	141
Wind-reliever series		Hold each pose of the series for at least six breaths. Repeat one time on each side.	Most people will benefit from using a strap for this series.	135
Savasana		Relax your breath and body. Hold for 5 to 10 minutes.	Use your props to make yourself comfortable and support your body. Add in a breathing exercise if desired.	152

Energizing Sequence IV: Half-Sun Salutation With a Chair

The sun salutation is probably the most popular and widely practiced sequence that exists. That's a big claim, but I feel pretty confident saying it! There are two classic versions of a sun salutation sequence, and both involve a lot of getting up and down off the floor. I find them to be inaccessible for lots of folks, and so I prefer to teach a version that creates much more space for people to find the benefits without engaging in the struggle! This sequence is performed from standing with your hands coming to a chair seat for stability and support. You can always substitute in a wall for a more supported option, or, if you're looking for an accessible challenge, you can explore options on the floor or with blocks in your hands. Try the sequence in many ways to experience all the variety available to you!

Props Needed

Chair

Blocks

Wall

Tips for Plus-Sized Bodies

As long as the chair you're using is sturdy and on a nonslip surface, you can trust it to hold your weight. Push the chair up against a wall for an extra feeling of support.

Pose	Photo	Pose notes	Pose options	Page
Mountain		Hold for two full breaths.	Step your feet wider for greater stability.	91
Forward-fold		Exhale into the pose and bring your hands or forearms to the chair seat. Hold for two to three breaths.	Step your feet wider apart to make space for your belly. Stay here longer if the pose feels extra good.	94
High-lunge		Inhale and step your right foot back into the lunge. Exhale and lift your chest and arms into a backbend. Hold for two breaths.	Practice low-lunge, page 80, with your foot on the chair or from kneeling for a different experience of the pose.	120

Pose	Photo	Pose notes	Pose options	Page
Downward-facing dog		Bring your hands to the chair seat, inhale, and step your feet back, shifting your weight into your legs. Hold the pose for two breaths.	Place your hands on the chair seat or move them to blocks on the floor or the floor itself.	96
Plank		Rise up on your toes and shift your hips forward to make a straight line from head to toe. You may need to adjust your hand or foot placement. Hold for two breaths.	Move to a wall for a more supported option. Move to the floor, with or without support, for an accessible challenge.	86
Downward-facing dog		Shift your weight back into the pose and hold for two breaths.	Place your hands on the chair seat or move them to blocks on the floor or the floor itself.	96
High-lunge		Inhale and step your left foot forward into the lunge. Exhale and lift your chest and arms into a backbend. Hold for two breaths.	Practice low-lunge, page 80, with your foot on the chair or from kneeling for a different experience of the pose.	120
Forward-fold		Exhale into the pose and bring your hands or forearms to the chair seat. Hold for two to three breaths.	Step your feet wider apart to make space for your belly. Stay here longer if the pose feels extra good.	94
Mountain		Hold for two full breaths.	Step your feet wider for greater stability.	91

Repeat the sequence again, this time bringing the left foot back into the lunge so the movements are even on both sides of the body. You can continue to repeat the sequence as many times as you like. One of the things I love about this sequence is that, once your body learns the movements, it becomes a moving meditation. You can practice this sequence any time you need fresh energy!

CONCLUSION

I hope you found some inspiration, energy, and motivation in the practices I've included in this chapter! I know how it feels to have low energy or be in a funk and want to do something about it, but, ultimately, it feels like it's too much work to take action. Whether you're feeling low, tired, or otherwise not great, there's something here to help you lift your energy level and maybe clear your head a bit. If you've tried a practice from this chapter, how did it go? Did your practice help you perk up at all? Did you learn any lessons about what is impactful for your mood or energy? Paying attention to these things over time can teach you a lot about how your brain and body work. You can even take notes to help you find patterns in your mood and behaviors. I've found that really helpful for me and learned that I tend to get tired at certain times and can plan my day to include a little energizing yoga to combat the afternoon fatigue.

Coming up in the next chapter are the sequences I designed to help you relax. I don't know about you, but I have anxiety and often need to use the yoga tools I have to help me find more peace and ease in my mind and body. I hope these can do the same for you. You can try them as is or use them as inspiration to experiment in whatever ways feel good to you. You're the boss of your body and of your practice! Remember that even just a few minutes of breathing, restorative poses, or gentle movement can make a big difference in how you feel. Bring that important question back to your mind when you're feeling short on time—what is the least I can do? The least you can do is powerful!

CHAPTER 10

RELAXING PRACTICES

Relaxing and calming yoga can be the perfect tool for the end of your workday, the beginning of a challenging week, or simply a stressful moment in your life. Whether you're in crisis or maintaining a healthy self-care practice, relaxation is important for your health and wellness. Remember to check in with your body and mind to ask what they need. Drink some water, take some deep breaths, and take a little time for a grounding yoga practice.

Throughout this book, we've explored a number of poses that lend themselves to a stress-relieving and relaxing practice. This chapter presents a number of sequences of varying lengths that I created to bring peace, ease, and calm into your day. The poses included are all explained in this book, so look out for the page numbers to refresh your memory about the benefits, alignment checklists, pose options, accessible challenges, and plus-size-specific tips. Take a look at the sequences included in this chapter to find what fits your needs best right now. There are sequences of different lengths and also options to incorporate standing, seated, and reclined poses.

While you practice these sequences, I want you to focus on letting go of the rest of your day. Keeping your to-do list, replaying an interaction over and over again in your mind, and thinking about what needs to be done are all things that will keep you from fully relaxing and getting the benefits of your practice. Allow yourself to acknowledge any thoughts that come up and then let them float away. You don't need to hold onto them during your practice! Turn off your phone and remove any distractions that might keep you from immersing yourself in these grounding sequences. Remember that you deserve these moments of peace and self-care.

Relaxing Sequence I: 10 Minutes

This seated and reclined practice is a 10-minute sequence to bring your focus from outside to inside your body. It's a great midday or afternoon practice to ground and refresh yourself for the rest of your day. Feel free to extend the length of your holds or stay in legs-up-the-wall for more time if you'd like to extend the length of this practice. All the poses in this sequence are seated or reclined, and you have the option of using a chair for support if you don't have a wall available.

Props Needed

Blanket

Wall

Strap

Tips for Plus-Sized Bodies

Move the belly to make space in these postures. Place a folded blanket under your sacrum or hips during legs-up-the-wall for a little padding.

Pose	Photo	Pose notes	Pose options	Page
Bound-angle		Begin with three deep, clearing breaths. Focus on grounding yourself and getting present in your body. Hold for 15 to 20 breaths.	If your hips or back are uncomfortable, you can adjust your legs to any seated position.	63
Cat–cow		Move with your breath between cat and cow pose. Take your time. Repeat 10 times.	Come to tabletop, page 65, and practice on hands and knees for a different option.	67
Supported fish		Come into the posture and hold for 15 to 20 breaths.	If this isn't comfortable for your body, come into any supported backbend and hold.	150
Legs-up-the-wall		Begin by holding the pose for 20 to 30 breaths. Change your leg position or continue to hold for another 20 breaths.	Practice the three-part breathing technique, page 56, as you hold the pose.	144

Relaxing Sequence II: 30 Minutes

This 30-minute sequence features standing, seated, and reclined poses to be performed using a chair for stability, support, and a fresh perspective on poses. The sequence can help to shift your mood and bring a calming energy into your day. It's a great bedtime practice to gently move and prepare your body for a restful night's sleep. You can even practice this next to your bed and then finish with savasana in bed so you can drift off to sleep easily!

Props Needed

Chair

Blanket

Blocks

Bed

Tips for Plus-Sized Bodies

Step your feet wide and bring your belly to the center to make space in the forward-folds.

Pose	Photo	Pose notes	Pose options	Page
Mountain		Take 10 deep breaths. Focus on grounding yourself and getting present in your body.	Inhale and raise your arms overhead. Exhale and lower your arms by your sides.	91
Forward-fold		Repeat six times, moving in time with your breath instead of holding in the folded position. Inhale and stretch up and then exhale and fold forward.	Widen your stance to make space for your belly. Practice these moving forward-folds from seated on a chair for more support.	94
Downward-facing dog		Raise and lower your heels or bend and straighten your knees. Hold for 15 to 20 breaths.	Keep your hands on the floor, on blocks, or on a chair seat. You can place your hands on your bed if you don't have a chair in your bedroom.	96
Cat–cow		Place your hands on a chair seat or bed top. Move with your breath between cat and cow pose. Take your time. Repeat 10 times.	Come to tabletop, page 65, and practice on hands and knees for a different option.	67

(continued)

Relaxing Sequence II: 30 Minutes *(continued)*

Pose	Photo	Pose notes	Pose options	Page
Five-pointed star		Focus on extending out in all directions. Hold the pose for 10 breaths.	Add slow and gentle side-bends for a nice torso stretch.	105
Forward-fold		Exhale into the pose and bring your hands or forearms to the chair seat. Hold for 10 to 15 breaths.	Step your feet wider apart to make space for your belly. Stay here longer if the pose feels extra good.	49
Downward-facing dog		Inhale and step your feet back to shift into the pose. Hold the pose for 10 breaths.	Alternate bending your knees or lifting your heels as you hold the pose.	96
Mountain		Take six deep breaths. Focus on noticing the sensations in your body and connecting with your breath.	Inhale and raise your arms overhead. Exhale and lower your arms by your sides.	91
Simple twist		Come to a seated position and practice the pose, moving gently with your breath, six times.	Add dynamic movement by moving in and out of the twist with each inhale and exhale instead of holding the pose.	70
Head-to-knee		Hold the posture for 8 to 10 breaths. Repeat two times on each side.	Make sure your hips are facing the front. Sometimes they shift when getting into the pose.	76
Reclining bound-angle		Come into the pose and hold for 20 breaths.	Use props under your knees for support and to relieve tension in your back and thighs.	147

Pose	Photo	Pose notes	Pose options	Page
Wind-reliever series		Hold each pose of the series for at least six breaths. Repeat one time on each side.	Most people will benefit from using a strap for this series.	135
Savasana		Relax your breath and body. Hold for three to five minutes.	Practice from a seated or a supine position. Use your props to make yourself comfortable.	152

Relaxing Sequence III: 30 Minutes

This 30-minute seated and reclined practice can be performed completely on the floor or while seated on a chair and reclined on the surface of your choice. I love to move to my bed for the reclined poses! Another great bedtime prep sequence, this one incorporates more of a restorative yoga feeling with fewer poses held for longer times. There's minimal movement and no standing, so try this sequence when you need major relaxation vibes!

Props Needed

Chair

Strap

Blocks

Blanket

Bolster

Tips for Plus-Sized Bodies

Move your belly to create space in many of these poses. Extend the length of your arms with blocks or a strap.

Pose	Photo	Pose notes	Pose options	Page
Bound-angle		Begin with three deep, clearing breaths. Focus on grounding yourself and getting present in your body. Hold for 10 breaths.	Begin in mountain, page 91, if practicing in a chair.	63
Wrist and hand exercises		Practice from any comfortable seated position.	Repeat again if desired.	44
Neck and shoulder exercises		Practice from any comfortable seated position.	Repeat again if desired.	46
Cat–cow		Move with your breath between cat and cow pose. Repeat 10 times.	Come to tabletop, page 65, and practice from kneeling for an accessible challenge.	67

Pose	Photo	Pose notes	Pose options	Page
Wide-leg forward-fold		Exhale in the fold and hold for three to five minutes. Bring your forehead to rest on a stack of blocks. Use this support to allow you to release fully into the stretch.	If practicing from a chair, rest your forehead on the wall or other support.	78
Supported bridge		Come into the pose and hold for 5 to 10 minutes. As you hold, practice the box breath technique, page 57.	Blocks will give a firmer support but can be uncomfortable for some. Try a bolster underneath instead.	141
Wind-reliever series		Hold each pose of the series for at least six breaths. Repeat one time on each side.	Most people will benefit from using a strap for this series.	135
Savasana		Relax your breath and body. Hold for 5 to 10 minutes.	Practice from a seated or a supine position. Use your props to make yourself comfortable.	152

Relaxing Sequence IV: 60 Minutes

This 60-minute sequence is a culmination of all the relaxing practices in this chapter. It begins with a few standing poses to get your body moving and then moves into seated and reclined postures to bring relaxation and ease into your day. There's a mix of stretching and resting postures to work out the kinks in your body and prepare you for meditation, bedtime, or just to relieve stress. Toward the end of the practice, there are some restorative yoga postures to hold for longer times. Sink into these and let them infuse your body with softness and ease!

Props Needed

Chair   Wall

Blocks   Blanket

Tips for Plus-Sized Bodies

Move your belly to create space in many of these poses. Extend the length of your arms with blocks or a strap. Push the chair up against a wall for an extra feeling of support.

Pose	Photo	Pose notes	Pose options	Page
Mountain		Take 10 deep breaths. Focus on grounding yourself and getting present in your body.	Inhale and raise your arms overhead. Exhale and lower your arms by your sides.	91
Forward-fold		Repeat six times, moving in time with your breath instead of holding in the folded position. Inhale and stretch up, exhale and fold forward.	Widen your stance to make space for your belly. Practice these moving fold forward from seated on a chair for more support.	94
Downward-facing dog		Hold for 8 to 10 breaths and then come to standing. Lift your heels one at a time and shift your hips side to side.	Keep your hands on the floor, on blocks, or bring them to a chair seat. Stay here longer if it feels particularly good.	96

Pose	Photo	Pose notes	Pose options	Page
Tabletop		Gently move your hips side to side or experiment with any kind of movement that feels interesting. Hold the pose for 10 breaths.	If your wrists are uncomfortable, come to a standing version of the pose with your hands on a chair seat.	65
Cat–cow		Move with your breath between cat and cow pose. Repeat 10 times.	Practice from a seated position if kneeling feels uncomfortable.	67
Reclining bound-angle		Begin with three deep, clearing breaths. Focus on grounding yourself and getting present in your body. Hold for 10 breaths.	Practice mountain, page 91, if practicing in a chair.	147
Wrist and hand exercises		Practice from any comfortable seated position.	Repeat again if desired.	44
Neck and shoulder exercises		Practice from any comfortable seated position.	Repeat again if desired.	46
Simple twist		Exhale into the twist and hold for six to eight breaths on each side. Repeat two times.	Add dynamic movement by moving in and out of the twist with each inhale and exhale instead of holding the pose.	70
Wide-leg forward-fold		Exhale in the fold and hold for three to five minutes. Bring your forehead to rest on a stack of blocks. Use this support to allow you to release fully into the stretch.	If practicing from a chair, rest your forehead on the wall or other support.	78
Ankle and foot exercises		Flex and point as fully as it feels comfortable. Be gentle if you're not warmed up.	Repeat again if desired.	45

(continued)

Relaxing Sequence IV: 60 Minutes *(continued)*

Pose	Photo	Pose notes	Pose options	Page
Supported fish		Come into the posture and hold for 5 to 10 minutes.	If this isn't comfortable for your body, come into any supported backbend and hold.	150
Legs-up-the-wall		Hold the pose for five minutes. Change your leg position or continue to hold for another five minutes.	Strap your legs together to relieve strain on your thigh muscles. Bring your legs to a chair for another option.	144
Supported bridge		Come into the pose and hold for 5 to 10 minutes. As you hold, breathe intentionally and notice all the sensations in your body.	Blocks will give a firmer support but can be uncomfortable for some. Try a bolster underneath instead.	141
Wind-reliever series		Hold each pose of the series for at least six breaths. Repeat one time on each side.	Most people will benefit from using a strap for this series.	135
Savasana		Relax your breath and body. Hold for 10 to 15 minutes.	Use your props to make yourself comfortable and support your body. Add in a breathing exercise if desired.	152

CONCLUSION

You made it! This is the last chapter in the book, and you've learned so much along the way. Your yoga toolbox is filled to the brim with breathing exercises, warm-up movements, and sequences with all types of poses. With this information, you're ready to incorporate yoga into your daily life in so many ways. I hope that the healing benefits of this practice can be a source of comfort, support, and growth in your life. I know we've covered a lot, but you have the rest of your life to soak up more and more information and nuance about the practice of yoga. I can't wait for you to keep learning and feeling how yoga can help you to shift the way you feel in your body and about yourself as a whole!

I hope this last chapter helped you get ideas and inspiration for adding more ease and gentleness into your days. These relaxing practices can be tailored to fit the different needs you have throughout your days and will always be here waiting for you. Don't forget that softness, gentleness, and ease are just as important as big energy and powerful movement. Practicing these relaxing sequences balances your body and your life. This balance is important! Use all the tools in your toolbox to create a harmonious yoga practice that enriches and bolsters your life. I know there's a lot of information and tips that have been thrown at you throughout this book. It may be helpful to keep a notebook where you can write down questions or things that need clarifying as you're practicing and applying yoga in your life. That way you can come back to the book and know what you're looking for. It's easy to forget a question or thought you had mid-practice! If nothing else, I want you to take to heart the following reminders:

■ Be gentle and patient with yourself. This world can make this challenging. As a plus-size person, you're taught that you take up too much space and that your ultimate goal should be to make yourself smaller, to minimize yourself and your needs. Remember that you're worthy of softness, kindness, gentleness, and patience. You deserve the grace and patience you treat others with, and there's no reason to deny yourself these things. Your yoga practice can be a balm on your heart as mine has been for me. There's so much healing to be found in yoga, and you deserve that. Please remember this when it seems like the world is saying otherwise.

■ Your yoga practice doesn't have to look like anyone else's. Yoga is not a competition. It isn't a one-size-fits-all type of practice. Everyone comes to yoga with different experiences, perspectives, trauma histories, abilities, and needs. Our bodies are different, and so our yoga is different. The same pose can look dramatically different depending on who is practicing. Please remember that your practice of the physical postures and all the other limbs of yoga doesn't have to look like anyone else's. Meditation doesn't have to be performed seated with legs tucked into complicated shapes and a Zen atmosphere. Your meditation might look like an intentional washing of dishes or a slow walk around a park. Your yoga practice is your own—no expensive leggings, headstands, or pretzel poses needed.

■ Your body is not a problem. Much of the rhetoric about yoga still affirms that larger bodies can't perform poses and need to modify what they're doing to get as close to the traditional form as possible. Honestly, this part of the yoga world is so disappointing to me! I want to remind you, in case this is the only place you're hearing it, that your body is not a problem. Please consider that yoga has changed dramatically over time as new populations found it and tailored it to their needs. We find ourselves in that changing space right now. Every year, more yoga teachers are understanding that accessibility and equity are important in getting the benefits of yoga to everyone. If you haven't been exposed to this changed perspective, you need to hear this the most. Your body is not a problem! The poses are adaptable to fit your needs, not the other way around. Yoga can be molded and adapted to your needs so that you can get all the healing benefits it provides.

■ You deserve the healing benefits of yoga as you are. So many of us who live in larger bodies have believed that we needed to wait to do the things we dreamed about until we achieved a body worthy of those endeavors. I fully understand what that feels like, and, if you do as well, I want you to know I see you. If you're still in this space of putting off until x, y, or z happens, please hear me when I say not to wait! What if you never lose weight and are plus size for your whole life? Will you forgo the pleasure, excitement, and fulfillment of whatever you're putting off? What would happen if you just allowed yourself to live fully the life you want?

Some plus-size folks tell me that they'll try yoga when they lose weight because they don't want to inflict their spandex-clad butt on anyone else. Or they wait because they fear being judged or seen practicing in a plus-size body. Y'all, I want to give you a big hug! I know what that feels like, and it sucks. I don't want to try and convince you to do something you aren't interested in or don't feel that you're ready to try. I do, however, want to encourage you to live fully the life you have now, in the body you have now. Having a larger body doesn't negate your worth. It doesn't mean you don't deserve to access the joy and embodiment to be found in a yoga practice. I hope you truly consider these words and know that I understand where you are and what you're thinking. I lived there for a really long time and know the changes that happened in my life when I allowed myself to take a chance and try. I say all of this because I want for you what I was able to find myself. There is so much healing and benefit to be had if you give yourself permission in the body you have right this moment.

I'm so honored to be your guide on this journey through the world of yoga! I hope you've felt seen and are excited to continue your yoga practice in your daily life. If you feel overwhelmed with all the information, remember that you can always press pause and come back later. Yoga will always be here for you, no matter if you've taken a break for 15 minutes or 15 years. It can be your constant companion and support system all in one. I'd like to conclude this book with a special mantra I wrote just for you. When you need some support, connection, or affirming thoughts, I hope this can make you feel loved and supported. Bring your hands to your heart and connect with your body as you repeat the following:

I honor the light within me and celebrate my strength and softness.

I give myself permission to try, to love, and to learn from my mistakes.

I celebrate my courageous heart and send gratitude to my body and mind.

I affirm that I am worthy of love and respect, from outside and from within.

ABOUT THE AUTHOR

Laura Burns is a Yoga Alliance Experienced Registered Yoga Teacher (E-RYT 200) and a certified provider of Yoga Alliance Continuing Education hours. She holds a certification with Curvy Yoga and is a certified instructor with Accessible Yoga and Punk Rock Hoops. She is a community partner with the Yoga and Body Image Coalition and the creator of the HoopAsana and Radical Body Love yoga philosophies and practices.

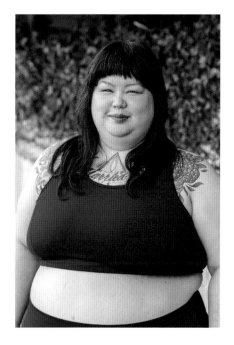

Burns is a leader in the world of plus-size yoga and has studied with a number of recognized experts in the field of size-inclusive yoga, including Anna Guest-Jelley (Curvy Yoga) and Abby Lentz (HeavyWeight Yoga). In addition to training with these mentors, she continues to attend workshops and trainings on a variety of yoga disciplines, teaching techniques, and innovations in props and support. She has been interviewed for or authored a number of magazine articles, blog posts, podcasts, and television spots.

Burns believes that every woman deserves to respect and honor the body she has today. Her personal mission is to help people be more present in their bodies and more loving toward themselves, moving forward toward advocating for themselves and living the life they deserve.

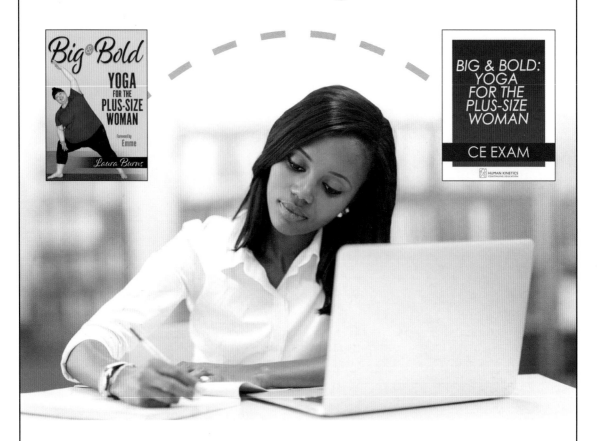
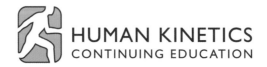